Fighting Childhood Obesity

I May Look Cute To You... But You Don't Know the Injustice You Are Doing to Me

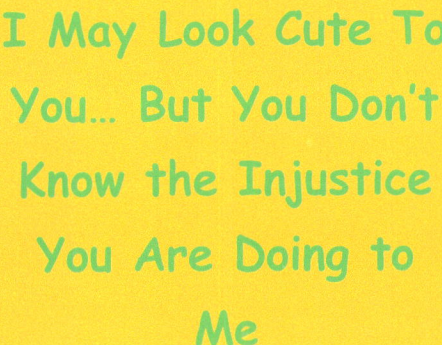

By:
Oliver Greene

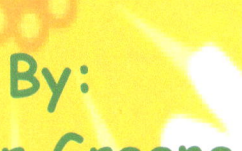
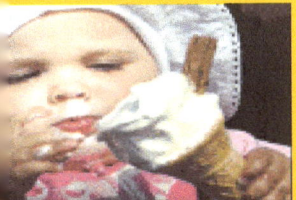
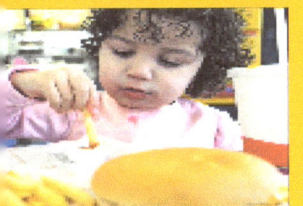
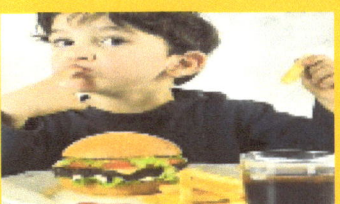
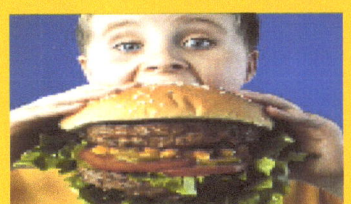
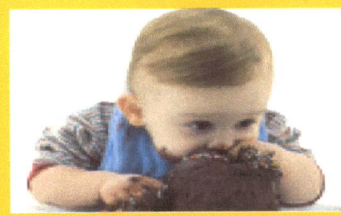
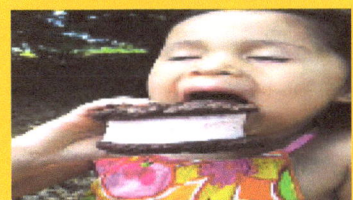
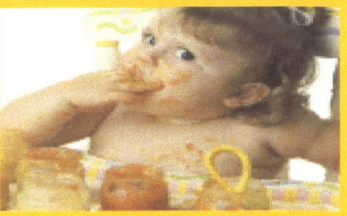
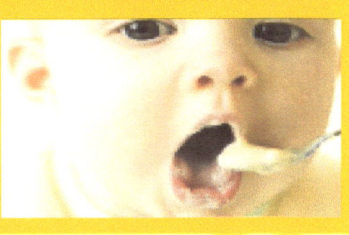

Contents

Introduction

The prevalence of obesity in children has ascended dramatically and at an alarming rate for the past several decades in the US. According to the American Academy of Paediatrics, the frequency of obesity and associated medical problems has reached an epidemic extent. Up to 30% of children and teenagers are already obese, while another 30% of this population is at great threat of becoming obese.

Obesity has become a very serious issue which can result in many physical and social consequences that carry on into adulthood. Therefore, it is important that we implement prevention programs and get a better understanding of childhood obesity. However, considering it a simple task would not be a wise step because the science behind childhood obesity is highly multifaceted and can differ between individuals. Common sense and medical advice are usually the most effective and safest ways of reducing childhood obesity.

Evaluation of the condition of obesity in adults and children is very important for several reasons. If you are well aware of such information, you will be in a better position to prevent diseases related to obesity. While hormonal and genetic causes of obesity are rare, they do necessitate consideration for prevention options in obese children.

Also you can take measures to save your child from the diminishing self-esteem resulting from obesity factors. Although childhood obesity may have negative consequences for childhood self-esteem, the magnitude and prevalence of this problem remains controversial.

Start the evaluation process to reach the root of the obesity in your child/children. This is important because by paying attention to how things around your child are, you can take better preventative steps to help your child. The presence of obesity in at least one parent significantly increases the risk that an obese child will become an obese adult. This will also give you a chance to look beyond your child to the rest of the people in your house.

As parents, we should always be concerned about our children's needs. They should be able to tell us their problems and we should be able to find solutions and remedies for their problems.

Communicate with your child and try to understand the reasons for his or her obesity. This way, implementing a change in their lives will become easier for you. Learn about their experiences to help them fight obesity and help them through this difficult phase.

What makes us victorious in the end is searching for a way that is actually practical. Being a parent, it is all in your hands. This book is written to help you evaluate, understand and prevent each and every aspect of the child obesity epidemic. After you've finished reading this book, I promise that you will be encouraged to make a difference in stopping this growing epidemic of childhood obesity in America and throughout the world.

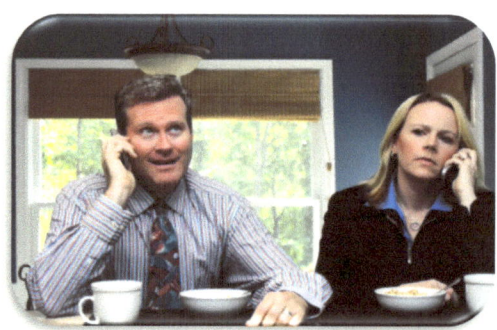

Health Choices – Do You Pay Attention to Your Child's Lifestyle?

Hey parents, if you ever had doubts that maybe it is your fault that your kids are fat, now there is even more proof that it is. In the past, I have embarrassed many parents for inflicting their lazy, poor, disgusting, obesity-inducing eating habits on their children. I have also taken notice of parents who are unaware of what is going on in their child's life and are busy with their hectic schedules.

According to statistics, there are two major reasons that cause childhood obesity. First, the parents of these obese children may be obese themselves. Second, the busy schedule of most parents does not allow them to pay attention to their children's lifestyle.

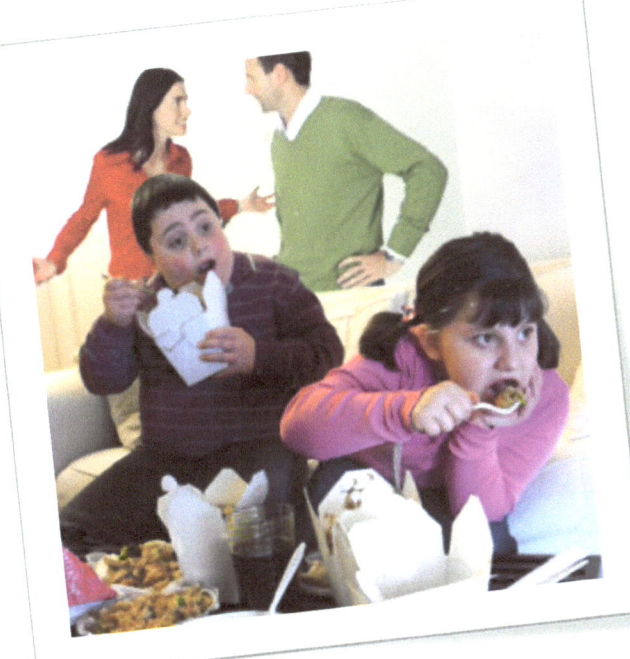

Having obese parents is indeed a genetic problem and cannot be overcome very quickly. However, it is not impossible either. Obese parents think that obesity cannot be cured by looking at themselves. But trust me, this is a complete myth. Obesity can be cured. Regardless of how busy parents are, they have to take out enough time for their children.

Obese parents must change the way they think. If they are still obese, it does not mean that there is no cure to obesity. It depends on how serious you take note of this growing epidemic. At least you can make efforts so it does not start in your home. Regardless of the fact that your child may be obese because of genetics, you can make a difference.

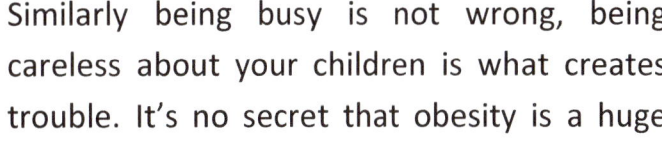

Similarly being busy is not wrong, being careless about your children is what creates trouble. It's no secret that obesity is a huge problem in America, and you might be among those people who do not understand the gravity of the situation. In fact, you may be contributing to this growing epidemic. Ask yourself: is there anything more important than your children's life? Perhaps not!

© Oliver Greene

In that case, does being busy seem to be a valid excuse? According to me, I don't think any excuse is valid enough to lead your child toward an unhealthy life. Obesity can lead to severe consequences if you fail to pay attention now.

Paying attention to your children's lifestyle does not mean you leave all your work and monitor your children. But taking a few hours off your busy schedule will definitely help your children. You must understand that your children need love, support and concern. And no one can do this job better than parents.

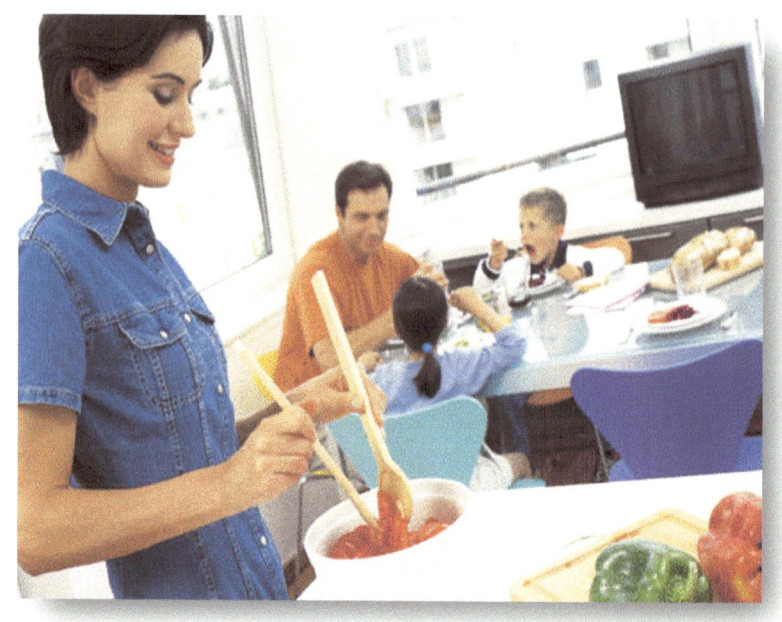

It is not mandatory that both parents should monitor children together. You can take turns to fulfil these responsibilities. This way you will also get time for your work and you don't have to worry about your children being on their own.

Children who are overweight or obese already have several emotional problems. At first you might face difficulty tackling your children because they are so used to being on their own. Bringing changes to their lifestyle all of a sudden may show some negative results in the beginning.

However, you should not get discouraged or disappointed. This is an expected reaction and your children have the right to do so. When children spend years taking decisions on their own, it is likely that any interference will be unwelcome.

The role of mother is however a major source of reliance when it comes to childhood obesity. Mothers who have jobs don't directly cause weight problems in their children, but busy families may accelerate weight gain by relying too much on frozen dinners and fast foods rather than preparing fresh, healthy meals.

In fact, I would say that it's not the parents' employment, but the environment. There needs to be improved access to healthy foods. Do not bring changes suddenly. This can be a shock for your children. Start with slow and steady changes until you reach the finish line!

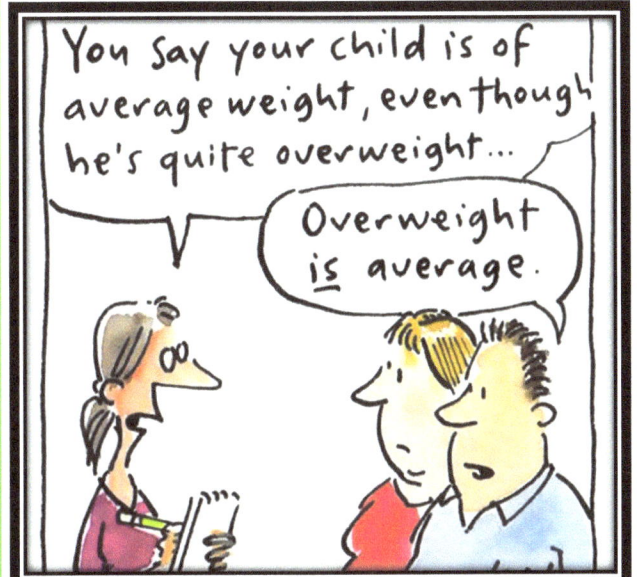

Obesity and Health Risks

First of all, parents should be aware if their children are overweight or obese. The biggest mistake many parents make, especially ones who are obese themselves is that they do not discourage their children from gaining more. In fact, they do not accept that their child is overweight in the first place. According to them, their child is normal and is living a healthy life. WRONG!!! This is the worst approach parents are taking against their children.

Find out if your child is obese and accept the truth so that you can start working on it before it is too late. Out of many issues that childhood obesity leads to, health risks is the major problem. Anything else can be ignored but this!

We all know that obesity can increase the possibility of certain serious diseases significantly. Many times, the seeds of obesity are sown in childhood, since significant weight gain as a child is often carried into adulthood.

However, this is not the only concern that exists with regard to childhood obesity. There are various adult diseases that are being reported in children and adolescents suffering from being overweight or obese. The incidence of such diseases was almost negligible among teens and children. This is why it is presumed that obesity is playing a major role in causing certain so-called "adult ailments" in America's youth.

Adult diseases in children can also occur due to environmental and genetic reasons. There has been a 400% increase in the number of obese children of ages six years and older in the last two and a half decades.

Obesity has severe health risks, which have been accepted by all experts. It exposes children to the following health problems:

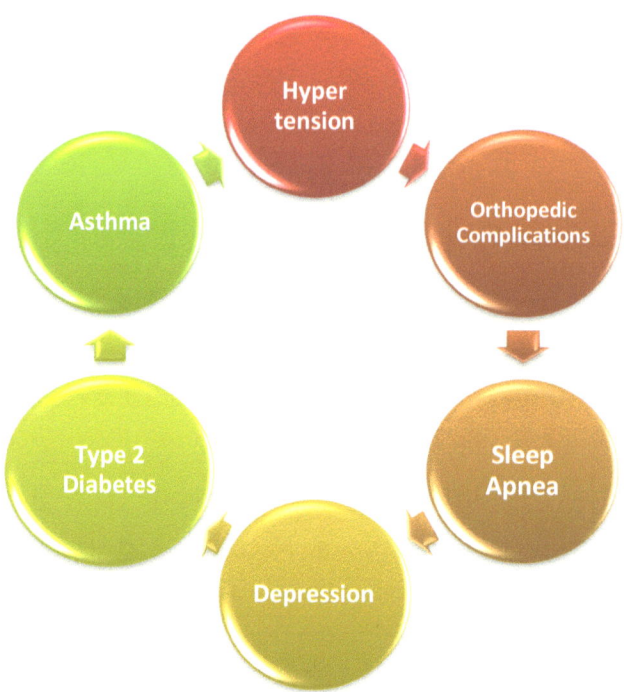

Hypertension – obesity leads to more frequent hypertension in children. It has been revealed that the frequency is around nine times more than usual.

Type 2 Diabetes – obese children, especially those with a family history of type 2 diabetes, run a significantly greater risk of developing the disease.

Orthopaedic Complications – the cartilage in lower joints and limbs in children is at the progressive stage. Since cartilage is unable to bear more than average weight, obesity can damage it to a great extent.

Sleep Apnoea – This is characterized as the absence of respiration and difficulty in breathing during sleep. This can cause a lot of trouble especially to little children.

Depression – the social and psychological stigma that is linked with obesity can be more traumatic during adolescence and childhood. This can lead to mental disorders such as depression.

Asthma – Many obese children are also at risk of developing asthma due to prolonged exposure to dust mites, lack of pulmonary exercise and other household allergens from leading a sedentary lifestyle.

Parents should encourage the thought of consulting their child's paediatrician to determine whether their child is obese. This is important because you have to first ascertain the weight gain due to the natural growth process of a child.

Apart from the common diseases mentioned above, there is a chance that your child

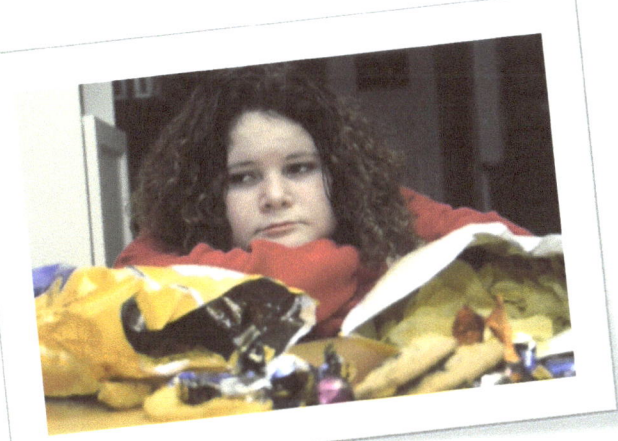

could be prone to many other much more dangerous diseases such as cancer, heart related diseases, high cholesterol, bone and joint problems, liver and gall bladder disease, low self-esteem etc.

Kids who are unhappy with their weight may also be more likely to develop substance abuse problems and eating disorders. Diagnosing and treating overweight and obesity in children as early as possible may reduce the risk of developing such severe medical conditions.

Another mental condition that children go through while facing obesity is low self-esteem. Obese girls and boys have significantly lower self-esteem than their non-obese friends during their childhood. According to research, it was also found that obese teens with esteem difficulties are more likely to engage in drinking alcohol and smoking. This is why; even doctors emphasize focusing on lifestyle issues for effective weight control rather than strict calorie counts and diets.

When it comes to childhood obesity, self-esteem and weight gain are like brothers. They are linked by one primary source, your confidence. If someone is low on self-esteem, it can cause this person to do many things that could affect their health. So what basically leads your children to low self-esteem?

Didn't you wish to become as thin and beautiful as your favourite model while you were young? Or didn't you fancy your favourite football player and wanted to play just like him/her? Even if you were unable to reach those goals, you have overcome it with time. But think about your children. Just wishing they were as good looking or active as their best friends is a natural part of growing up.

But learning what they can or can't change about their bodies and appearances is a part of growing up too. This can be really disappointing and can hit your child's self-esteem.

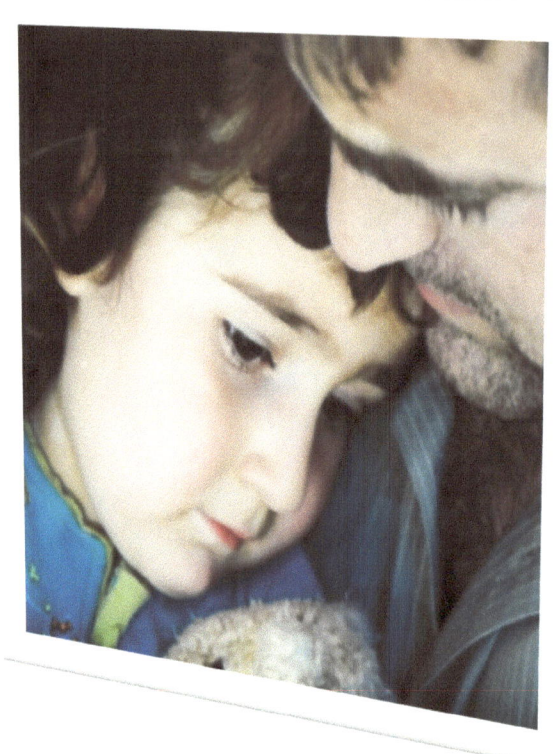

Regardless of what your children's weight is and how they feel about it, let them know you are there to help them be happy and healthy and that your love them a lot.

So what's your role? What can you do to boost the self-esteem and confidence in your little one again? There is so much you can do... so read on until you find out.

Physical Effects of Childhood Obesity

Do you know your child's weight? Have you been watching your child's weight to make sure that he or she is not putting on excess weight? Is your child physically active like his or her other friends?

Childhood obesity can lead to severe results in addition to those mentioned above. A person's bones are not fully formed until he or she reaches the late teenage years. When a child is obese or overweight, bone growth is affected because of all the extra weight.

The excessive stress on the child's bones hinders normal childhood growth and development. According to the United States Bone and Joint Initiative, the frequency of childhood obesity related joint and bone problems are at their peak.

To cut it short, excessive weight makes it difficult for bones to grow properly. This leads to joint problems that trouble the child throughout his or her life. As people age, pains and aches becomes a part of life. No parent wants their child to suffer an adulthood of crippling pain.

In some extreme cases, excessive weight results in Blount's Disease in children. When a young child is affected with Blount's, the position of leg bends inwards causing the shin to develop incorrectly. This can have long lasting ramifications and can progressively get worse. The child may further suffer the burden of wearing braces or have surgeries

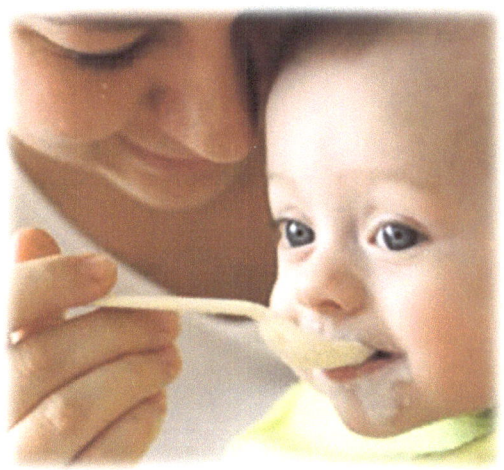

to overcome the problem. But don't you think you will be in a much better position if all you have to do is maintaining your child's healthy weight?

The global epidemic of childhood obesity can have a devastating impact on a child's musculoskeletal system. The body's building blocks are healthy bones and joints. The extra weight of the body pressurizes the body's building blocks causing problems in the growth and development of your child.

Parents now seem to have a better understanding that childhood obesity can lead to many diseases such as diabetes and heart problems. However, parents are still overlooking the potential effects of obesity on their child's bones, muscles and joints.

Arthritis, Blount's Disease and cartilage deterioration are severe and painful problems. The worst fact about the pain is that it makes the child even more reluctant to participate in physical activities. This makes it likely that the child will grow even more overweight.

You must take control of your child's weight immediately. The sooner the better.

The usual behaviour of parents towards children approaching junk food as snacks and meals is to give into their child's plea to make them happy. Just for the sake of their happiness and temporary satisfaction, this behaviour of parents often leads to allowing the child to choose his or her own menu. Sometimes parents give in because it is easier than saying no.

But parents must realize that their children are too young to understand the consequences of such decisions. For younger children, twenty-five is an older age. However, they still do not understand the concept of the pain they might face in their 30's, 40's and beyond because of the choices they make today.

You must take the responsibility of making decisions on behalf of your children for their good. Moreover, do not hesitate to say NO, when NO is what should be said.

Causes of Childhood Obesity

What are the causes of childhood obesity? Why is our child getting fatter day by day? Is my child suffering obesity?

There are several factors that lead to childhood obesity. However, blaming one specific behavior as the major cause of obesity in children is impossible due to the interactions they have with each other. There are many factors typically working in combination. Some are flexible to change while others are not. Sometimes unnecessary weight gain is caused by certain medical conditions such as genetic syndromes, endocrine problems and medications.

Even though there are some environmental and some genetic causes of childhood obesity, it is vital to know that weight gain, whether leading to severe or mild clinical obesity has several causes centering on an inequity between calories burnt in physical activity and calories consumed from food and drinks. Hence, unhealthy eating habits, lack of physical activity, or a combination of two are general causes of childhood obesity along with lifestyle and genetics, both playing a vital role in determining a child's weight.

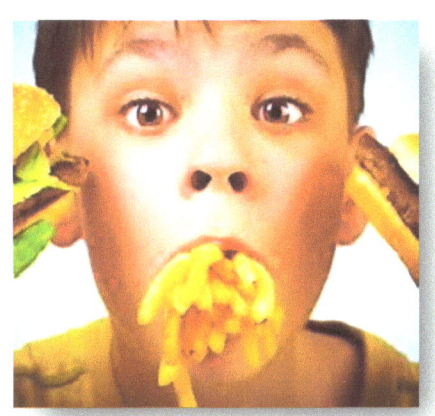

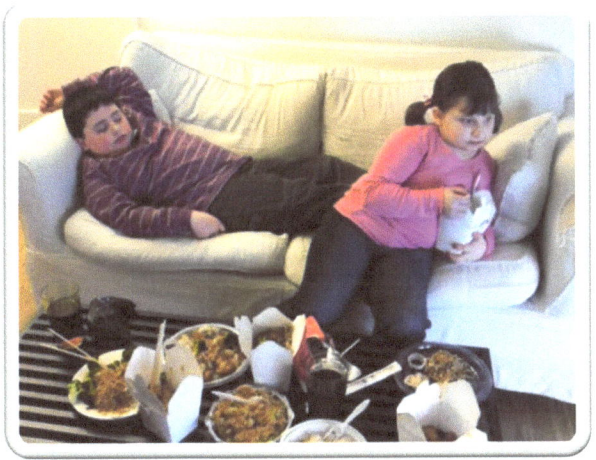

Considering the environment, it is another factor that is having a direct impact on a child's weight. The people around and their environment have a significant affect on the lifestyle and habits of little children. This is quite obvious because children will adopt things they experience in their environment and will follow the attributes of people around them.

Want to know the other contributing factors? Read On!

The Role of Food Marketing

For the first time in modern history, our **children's life expectancy could be lower than our own**. The reason: **obesity**. One culprit recognized is the commercialism to which children are exposed almost every day. Just like obesity, this food marketing will only increase if proper measures are not adopted to stem it now.

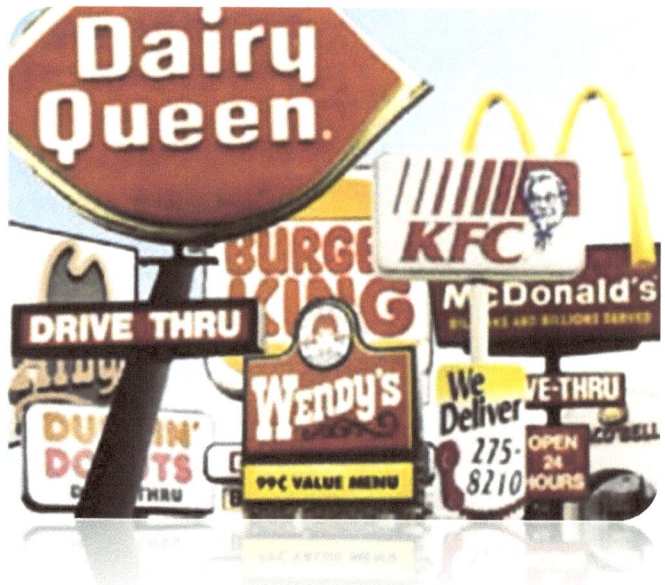

Food companies have bombarded the television with advertisements that are often promoting products that are harmful to health. According to Dale Kunkel, Communication professor at University of Arizona, the average child is exposed to around 40,000

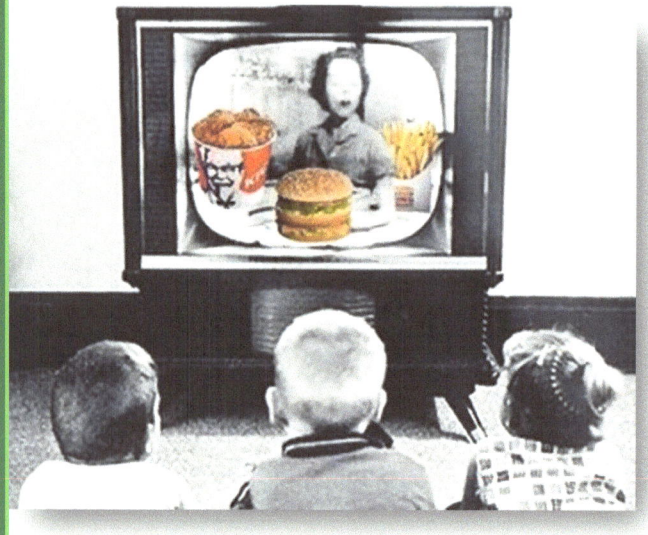

commercials on television alone each year. He also stated that the majority of these advertisements are targeted towards promoting candies, soda, sugared cereal and fast food.

While you may become the victim at the cash register paying the price for all of this advertising, your children will be paying the actual cost with their health. The role of fast food marketing in the childhood obesity problem is significant. Fast food restaurants are setting their marketing campaigns aggressively in order to target vulnerable groups. They are ready round the clock to serve you child with their not-so-healthy options on the menus.

Almost every day fast food dominates the headlines and has become a daily topic in the news. Whether it is because of their negative health effects (such as diabetes), low nutrition ingredients (such as Trans fats), or being linked to obesity.

Food marketing and obesity are linked. Since food companies are getting more aggressive in targeting kids, the entire world, especially America has experienced a rise in obesity. In fact, food marketing is targeting one out of four kids at a burger joint every day. Food marketing and obesity are so cohesive because they are designed to be. This fast food contains ingredients that make it addictive and induce hunger. It steals your health, energy, and directly causes obesity. This is why, the relationship between food marketing and obesity can't be ignored.

No doubts, these food marketing advertisements are so tempting and eye-catching that sometimes you can't even ignore them. Therefore, children should not be blamed. Although you cannot do anything about these advertisements, except for reducing the screen time for your children.

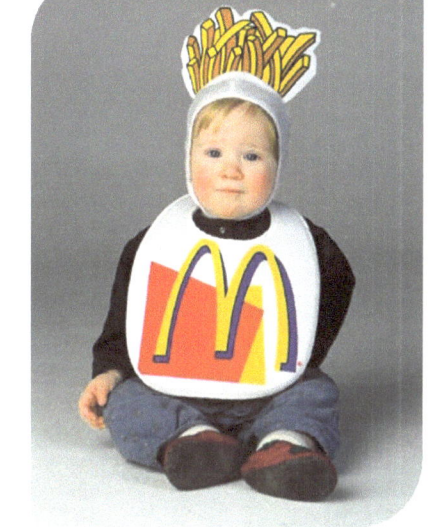

Moreover, do not always agree to what your children ask for. Fast food contains additive ingredients that may cause addiction. There is a chance that your little one might end up being addicted to fast food. Therefore, implement your measures before it is too late.

Are you still not sure how to prevent influential food advertising having an impact on your child? We have a solution for you right in this book. So carry on!

The Gaffe of Bad Food Combinations

Right when you are not paying attention, fast food companies speak to your children. Fast food is the most unhealthy food product marketed to children, other than sugar-sweetened beverages, and is aggressively and persistently targeted towards children starting as young as age two.

So what is food marketing actually doing?

© Oliver Greene

The fast food industry is spending over $4.2 billion dollars on different media advertisements. They are doing this to spread the word about their unhealthy yet tempting and delicious menus to little children who they are sure would love it.

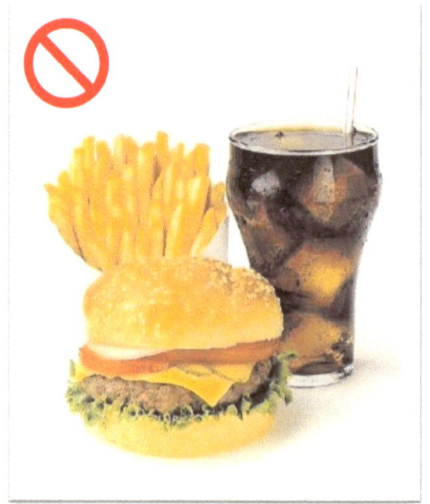

Some fast food advertisements appeal specifically to children. Characteristics of these ads include fun messages, kid's meal promotions, movie tie-ins and licensed characters. Not only are these advertisements a great turn-on for children, they will also force you to give them a treat at that particular restaurant the very same day.

So should you instantly agree to their wish or be reluctant about it? You should immediately say NO as soon as you hear such a plea. This book is not written to demote fast food restaurants but to promote your child's health. There are valid reasons why fast food is considered unhealthy for your children.

Branding is prominent in child-targeted ads, while food is not. When it comes to food, most restaurants feature their menu. However, the fact is that these restaurants use cheap combinations of foods without paying attention to its nutritional factors.

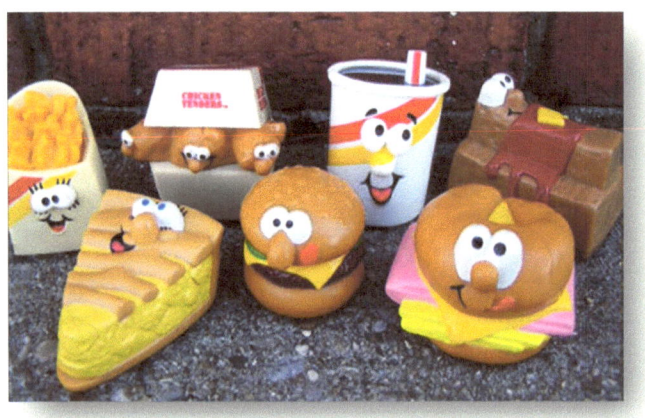

According to statistics, out of their 3000 different food combinations, only 0.05% has any nutrient for our children.

Although the growing epidemic of obesity is a problem for all, the fast food industry seems to only play the negative role. Their rich calorie food is what they are feeding your children in excess, resulting in your children becoming obese. The food prepared contains negligible amounts of nutrients required by children, making the food a complete waste in terms of nutrition for your children.

I wouldn't call this the mistake of the fast food industry. It is in fact your biggest gaffe. Being a parent, you must know the nutritional needs of your little ones. Moreover, you must also realize that these popular fast food restaurants are not fulfilling the nutritional requirements of your children. Instead, they are only helping to making your children overweight and obese.

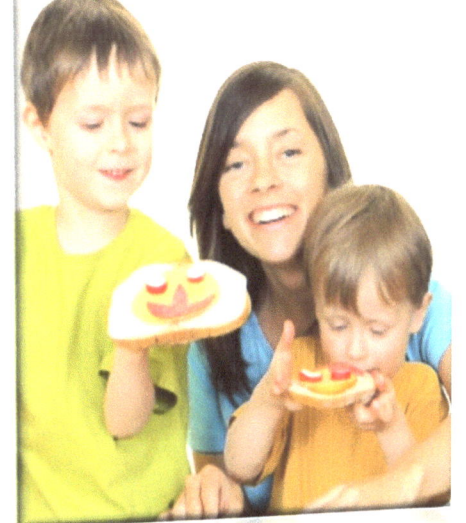

Stop your children from frequently requesting trips to fast food restaurants that engage in the most child-targeted advertising. Ignore such demands until you are able to control them. Make them a similar meal at home with more nutrition in it. Surprise them with the additional tie-ins these restaurants offer to grab children attention by purchasing them separately. But do not give in easily. You definitely don't want your child to continue to be a part of the severe growing epidemic of obesity.

Do not let these food marketing strategies dominate your little one like it dominates the headlines every other day.

The Contribution of Diet

Everyone agrees on the fact that children are becoming obese, but not everyone agrees on the causes. There are several reasons how childhood obesity and diet are proportional to each other in influencing child obesity. Our children are regularly consuming higher calories than they are burning through physical activities. However, this energy imbalance is resulting from their environment in neighbourhoods, schools and most importantly at home.

Around 60 per cent of the youth in the United States consumes high calorie fattening food that gradually leads to increasing weight and eventually results in childhood obesity and its related health issues. The remaining 40 per cent follow the suggested diet that includes minimum five servings of vegetables and fruits per day.

The US dietary patterns have taken a U-turn over the past few decades. The excessive nutrition has changed to under-nutrition as serious nutrition related problems are faced by both children and adults. Regardless of the fact that percentage of calories have turned down from total fat over the past thirty years, total calories have increased. Moreover, Americans are getting fonder of soft drinks day by day due to which they are gaining more calories and fewer nutrients.

There is in fact a significant reason behind the changes in the pattern of US dietary requirement. The reason is that eating habits have also changed drastically. Proper timely family meals are converted into continuous munching available for children to fill up on. Moreover, the busy schedules of parents have also forced children to look for their own diet in unhealthy snacks that are rich in calories. Furthermore, our environment also encourages children to consume large oversize meals at restaurants.

These are some of the major tendencies that are playing a vital role in increasing the rate of childhood obesity together with lack of physical activity and exercise.

Many kids just like to eat fast food from restaurants instead of eating healthy foods with vitamins and nutrients, whereas to fulfil the body requirements of essential vitamins and nutrients, kids must consume fresh vegetables and fruits.

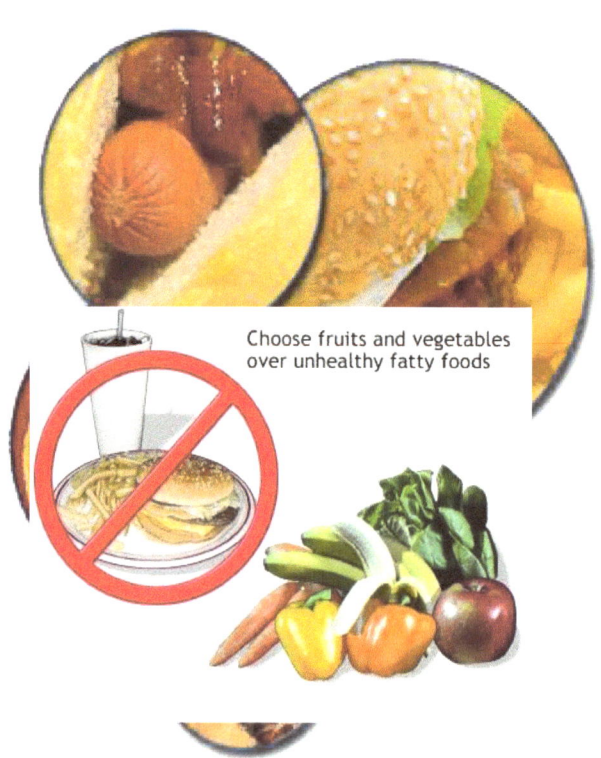

Choose fruits and vegetables over unhealthy fatty foods

Energy Imbalance

There are times when unhealthy food is the only factor held responsible for childhood obesity. To some extent, this statement is correct but the proper way to portray this in simple terms would be that childhood obesity is a result of energy imbalance. This means that the energy consumed is more than the energy used.

This imbalance occurs when a child consumes extra calories but is unable to burn it off through exercise or physical activities. These extra calories then make a permanent place in your body as fats, instead of being utilized as energy by consuming it. This will end up making major and prolonged changes in the body starting from weight gain and eventually turning into child obesity.

- The best definition of a calorie is a unit of energy supplied by food. A calorie is energy regardless of its generation source. Whether you are consuming fats, carbohydrates, proteins or sugar, all of them contain calories.
- Energy balance is like a scale. To maintain an efficient balance of calories in order to maintain your ideal body weight, the calories consumed must be balanced by the calories burned by exercise or normal physical effectiveness.

In the past, when food shortages were a common trend faced by our early ancestors, they introduced some alarming physiological processes that supported slowing down weight loss.

One of these protective mechanisms was to store the excess body fat that was utilized when food was scarce. In this age, however, we do not have to face the same food scarcity problems like our ancestors – thanks to the development of food production processes.

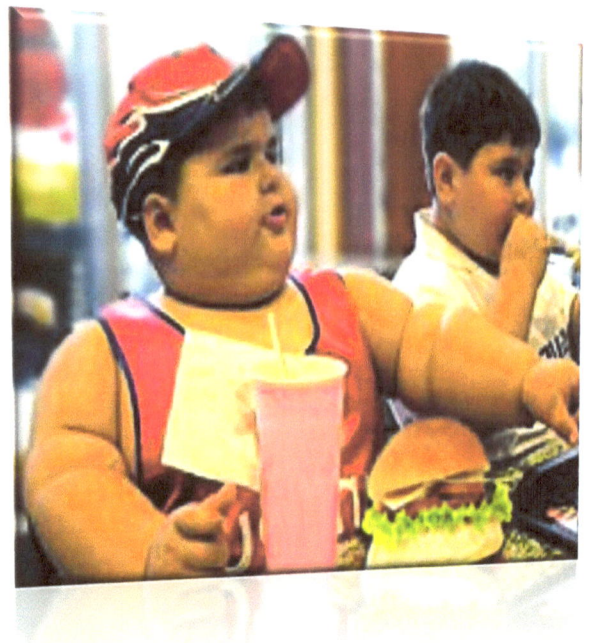

These same manufacturing processes that helped in increasing food shelf life along with increasing the amount of food available to us are also responsible in eliminating the healthy nutrients such as vitamins and fibre and leave the tasty sugars, fats and salts in place. To conclude children and obesity with less physical activities and exercise every day is due to technological advances and not food shortages any longer. The accumulation of such energy imbalance day after day is resulting in increase in childhood obesity.

Facts are incomplete on dietary patterns or a particular food that contributes towards unnecessary consumption of energy in teens and children. Eating meals away from home, large portion sizes for food and drinks, consumption of beverages having high calorie and high sugar and regular snacking on energy-dense foods increases childhood obesity.

Children may not be prepared to compensate timely meals for the excessive calories they have already consumed through sugar-sweetened drinks. However, the impact may be different considering different age groups of children. Liquid forms of energy may be less satiating than solid forms and lead to higher calorie intake.

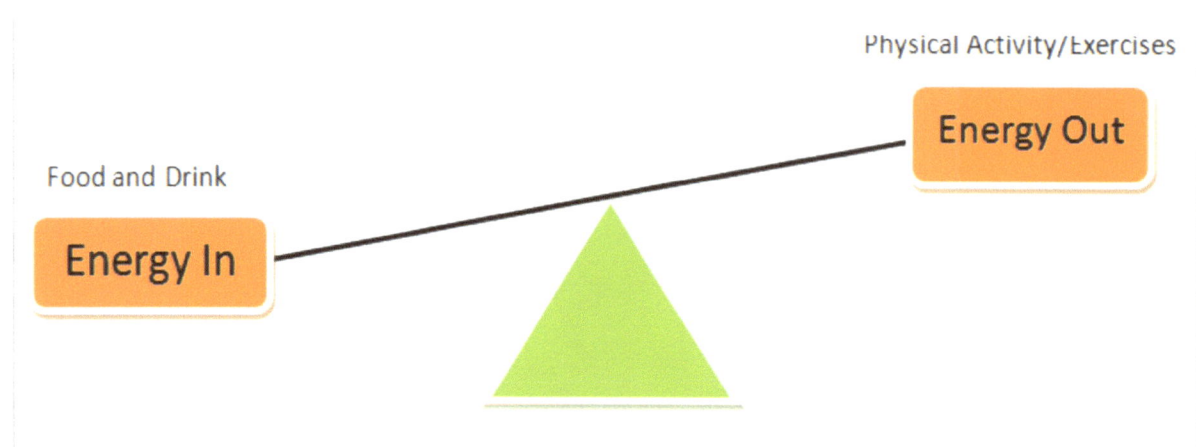

With these increases in weight will come increased health problems, which are a serious health risk not only for children but for adults as well. This makes it a complicated health concern to deal with. Environment and genetics may increase the risk of childhood obesity.

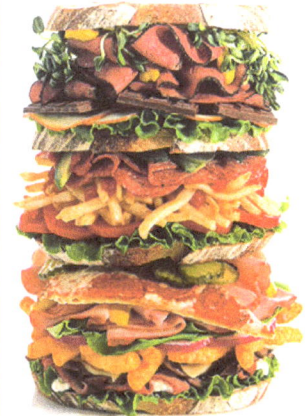

To sum it up, there is a selection of factors that play a role in childhood obesity. The behaviour of children towards physical activity and eating along with the environmental influence, play a fundamental role in creating an impact on childhood obesity which are indeed the greatest areas of treatment and prevention actions.

Obesity in Children and Nutritional Patterns

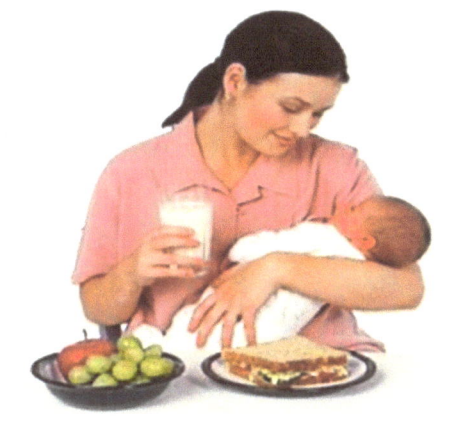

Wrong nutrition patterns and childhood obesity are strongly connected, resulting in several health issues related to obesity. Adolescents and children prefer to eat salty, sugary and saturated fats instead of nutritionally rich fruits and vegetables. Attention has also been grabbed by children focusing more on consuming unhealthy soft drinks and fast foods. The problem is even worse for those children who are prone to obesity genetically.

Families who have limited sources of income also experience inadequacy to access healthy food and this makes it even more difficult to construct a better and healthier diet. There is rising confirmation that the reason why adults are more susceptible to diseases is because they lack proper nutrition in early childhood. Therefore involving your child at an early stage will be a good way to start lessons.

Considering the alarming situation of childhood obesity, the need for adopting regular physical activity and healthy eating in children has never been greater. In the last three decades, the numbers of obese children have tripled respectively showing the lack of observation of busy-scheduled parents and continuation of poor eating habits.

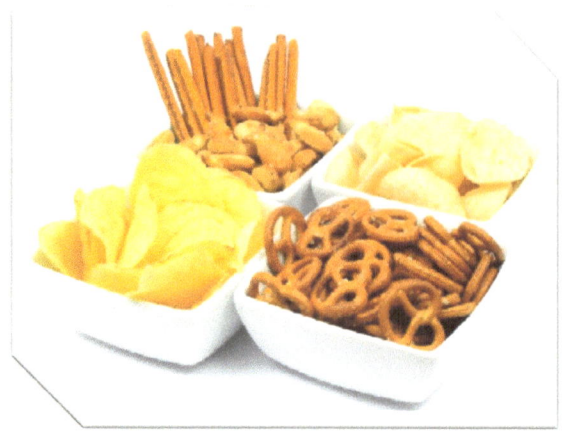

Poor eating habits include insufficient fruit, vegetable and milk intake while consuming excessive calories snacks. As far as calories are concerned, grain products are the highest calorie provider at the rate of 31 percent of daily consuming excessive calories. As far as calories are concerned, grain products are the highest calorie provider at the rate of 31 per cent of daily calories. Next are other foods, which have limited nutritional value of 22 per cent of daily calories. Different snacks account for 27 per cent of daily calories, which is higher than calorie intake at breakfast time (18 per cent) and at lunch time (24 per cent). However, it is still lower than dinner time calories (31 per cent).

For a child (age four and above), more than 41 per cent of daily snack calories come from other foods such as chocolates, chips, soft drinks, sweets, fruit drinks, preserves, syrup, oils and fats.

Parents are children's ideal and, therefore, they try to follow their parents in every manner. Even the food choices and habits are developed by seeing their parents and getting influence. Other sources of influence are friends, caregivers, schools, marketing and most importantly, technology and media. Let's see these sources in detail.

Blaming the Inactive Lifestyle

Did you know?

- One out of every three children (ages 2-19) in America is suffering obesity
- Obesity is causing around 112,000 deaths every year in the US

- One out of every three children born in the year 2000 are at a high risk of developing obesity and diabetes during their life
- Childhood obesity health issues are incurring around $3 billion/year in medical costs

Have you ever considered that there could be causes, other than food that can cause such alarming conditions in our countries and within our homes? Well there are! As mentioned in the last topic, inactive lifestyle is playing its role in increasing this growing menace. But there are other factors that help in creating a sedentary and inactive lifestyle. One such factor operating behind childhood obesity is **Media**.

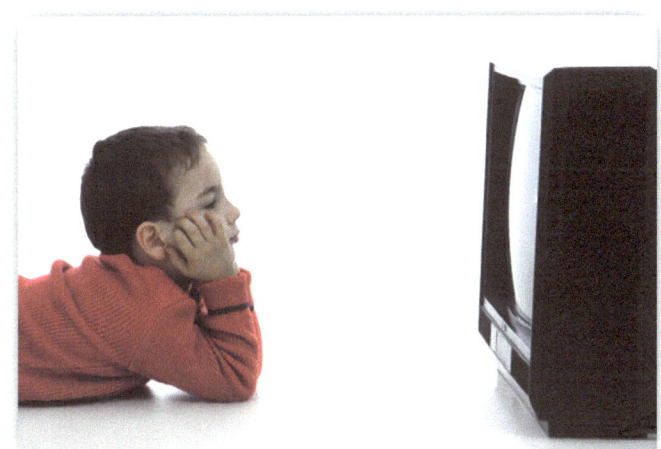

The Role of Media

According to several studies, it has been concluded that a kid's weight starts to increase in accordance with the number of hours the child is spending watching TV every day. Today, the growing statistic of childhood obesity is giving America great concern with regard to the health condition of its youth. The American Academy of Paediatrics (AAP) suggests that the screen time for children should be minimized to not more than two hours a day. However, many children have a TV set in their own room because of which the average hours a child watches TV falls between three to five hours each day.

Media is a significant source operating behind childhood obesity. Children are spending a considerable part of their everyday schedule with media. Children and teens who are fond of watching TV and are spending a substantial amount of time watching their favourite programs tends to be overweight or obese. This is not only because there is an imbalance in energy and less energy is spent, but also due to mindless eating and consumption of calorie rich foods.

There are logical factors behind blaming television as the major source behind sedentary lifestyle, excessive eating eventually resulting in obesity. Read on to find out why obesity is progressing in your child(ren).

- Dislocation of exercise and physical activity. Media engages the child's time that he could have used exercising or involving in different physical activities like playing and running. In short, the major emphasis is not on what the child is engaged in but rather what the child could have done if he/she was not watching TV.

- Television and other medias such as radio, magazines etc - are the main source of attractive food marketing advertisements that can build the urge for eating high calorie fast foods in the child. Most of the foods advertised on media belong to the category of fattening foods and therefore are rich in calories and unhealthy for children. Sugared cereals, candy bars and many more like such are some examples of unhealthy food choices made by children after watching those targeting advertisements.

- Because media does not require energy, there is a likelihood that your child will end up decreasing the resting metabolic rates as well.

- Media influences the intake of excess food because children eating while watching TV or playing games do not realize the quantity of food they are eating. This mindless eating is never healthy for young children and usually results in overweight or obesity.

Several studies were dedicated to finding out the connection between childhood obesity and media. Moreover, several experimental studies that held the agenda of decreasing media and screen time have also been completed lately. All the research did not conclude on the direct effects of reducing media time alone. However, according to the final report it is suggested that reducing media impact and screen time from our children's life will help in decreasing the risk of childhood obesity.

Not only television, other media sources such as internet, video games and even magazines are also contributory factor of continuous increase in weight. These days social media entertainment is one of the favourite leisure time activities for many children between the ages of ten to nineteen. Children spend time sitting in front of their computer screens and

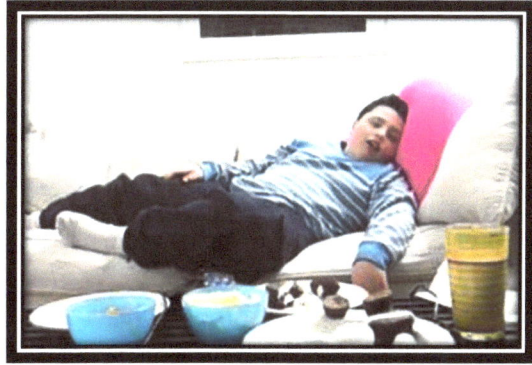

carelessly spend hours engaged in surfing. This way they are unable to spend time in daily physical activities or regular exercise schedules. Eventually, they adopt the sedentary lifestyle and learn to live with their obese bodies instead of making an effort.

Being engaged with media constantly is one of the major causes of childhood obesity. Sitting in a solitary position, without exercise and movement - results in increased body fat.

Some Facts…

> As concluded by the National Institutes of Health, children who spend more hours watching TV have the greater chances of suffering childhood obesity and its related health issues.
> The fame of video games, computers and media transform into an ever more sedentary lifestyle for many American children.
> On average children spend approximately three hours watching TV per day. Television not only supports mindless and continuous snacking but also encourages inactive and sedentary lifestyle.
> Last but not the least, only a minority of school children (one in five) is a regular participants of sports or other physical activities while the rest are spending the same time engaged in different media related entertainments.

Been engaged with media constantly is one of the major causes of childhood obesity. Sitting in a solitary position, without exercise and movement - results in increased body fat.

Technological Impact – Positive or Negative?

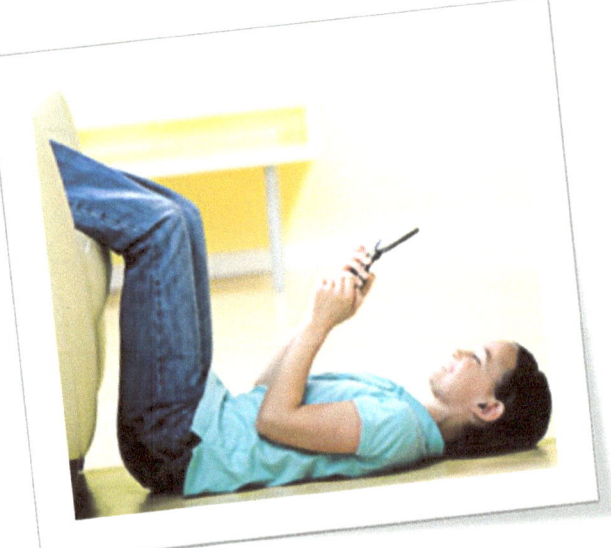

Technology! Sounds good until you are aware of the role it is playing in bringing your children to the threats of obesity. Technology is considered a culprit behind children and adults becoming fat.

Comparing whether those double sized fast food meals were the most evident reason of obesity or the double dose of innovation – no difference!

According to different researchers, sixty per cent of the excessive weight carried by obese children and adults is a result of the decline in the demand of physical work brought about by the advent of latest technology innovations. The remaining forty per cent however is a result of technological advancement made to the agriculture industries that has driven down real food costs.

Therefore, technology is considered to be a major contributor to these rising rates of obesity that also encourages sedentary behaviour in children. The ease of life provided by technological advancements is not only making children inactive but is also encouraging parents and other adults to follow the same trend.

Despite the fact that technology provides convenience, value and entertainment, it should not be replaced with the active play and movements in a child's life. Moreover, many researches pointed out that in past decades, demanding jobs meant that workers were in effect paid to exercise. Now workers with more sedentary jobs pay to exercise at the gym.

Thanks to modern technology, children are leading increasingly sedentary lifestyle and therefore are becoming a part of the growing problem in our society today. Children find it useless to walk all the way to talk to their friends when they have the facility to sit at home and keep up with them through texting or chatting? Neither do they feel the need to go out and play games when they have all the latest games right at their fingertips.

While technology makes our life easier, this is not an indication of making our life sedentary. Instead, modern technologies should be balanced with physical activity in order to keep our children healthy and free from obesity threats.

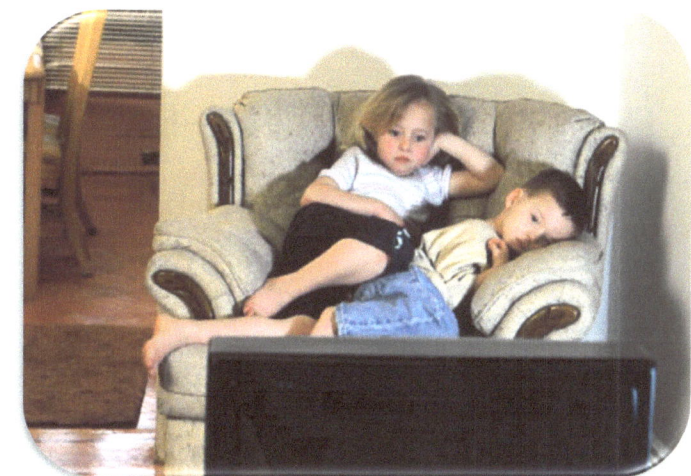

As soon as our children find us busy, they start to get more dependent upon 'electronic babysitters' also known as the TV and computer. Plus, even we feel easier knowing that our children must be enjoying their screen time and we can spend our time doing the things we need to do.

Don't let technology take over the physical activities of your child. Spending hours and hours in front of computers and TV and even eating at the same time does not only lead to childhood obesity but also contributes to continuing overeating in life as well.

It is strange how technology is having an adverse effect on the lives of our children. By implementing a few small changes you can make a big difference between bad habits caused by technology that are likely to lead to obesity and a healthy lifestyle.

We must remember that our children are our future and not machines. Therefore, it is our responsibility to counsel them and teach them good habits to carry with them all their lives.

School-Based Initiatives

According to research held in several schools in America, it is found that children who regularly eat school lunch have around 30 per cent higher chances of gaining more weight and becoming obese than those who bring lunch from home.

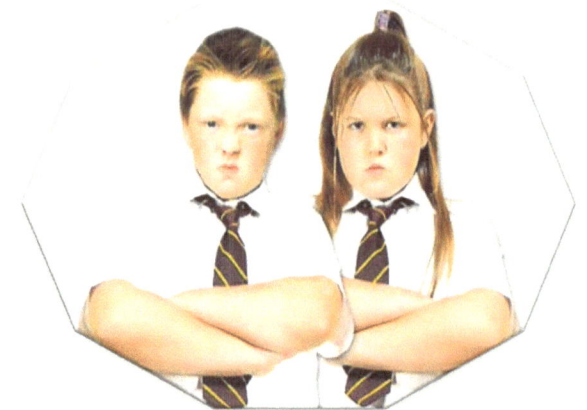

Children spend a large part of their life in school. In fact, most of the day is also spent at school and therefore children tend to adopt the lifestyle and behaviour choices from their early age. This is why, school life is considered to play a major role, even associated with obesity development during school age years.

A child's body weight is determined depending on the food intake and physical activity at school to a major level. By providing physical activity, healthy meals and adequate education, school guiding principles can play a vital role in preventing childhood obesity.

It is quite obvious that schools with environments that do not promote physical activity habits, healthy nutrition and health education are the dominating factor behind childhood obesity.

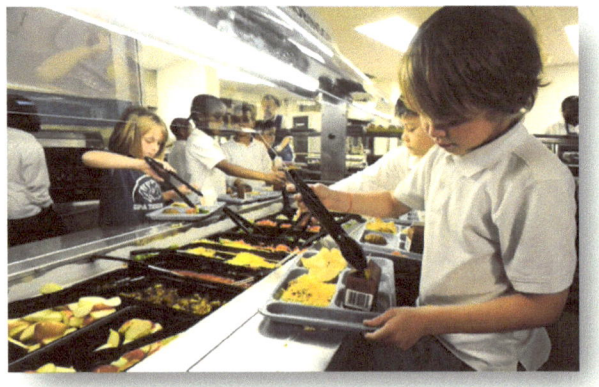

Usually, students are offered free or discounted meals in schools which leads to excessive intake of food among children. These programs may compose more than half the daily calorie intake for children who participate in those programs – especially those children who belong to low-income families.

However, the saturated and total fat content of meals that are offered by many schools exceed the limit required by children. Food preparation staff should be well trained in accordance with the obesity problem in children without lessening student participation rates.

Many schools also have student stores, snack bars, and vending machines that provide different types of food that are high in sugar and fat content. Students at schools which offer food sources free of cost or at discounts are less likely to consume juices, fruits, and vegetables than they need.

Schools that ignore the importance of physical activity are also held responsible for contributing in the growing epidemic of childhood obesity. This is because such schools do not encourage students to get involved in physical activity, resulting in these children gaining weight and becoming obese.

A national survey documented poor eating behaviour among American children. The results showed that only 21.4 per cent of school students are following proper nutrition, i.e. five servings per day of vegetables and fruits. 9.2 per cent reported using diet pills that were not prescribed by a physician; 13.5 per cent reported fasting for more than 24 hours in order to lose weight, while 5.4 per cent reported using laxatives and vomiting to control growing weight.

In another national survey, fat comprised an average of 35 per cent of total caloric intake in youth aged two to nineteen years, and almost two-thirds of these youth did not follow the recommended amount of fruits and vegetables required.

Many schools do not pay attention to giving their students adequate nutritional education to enable them to make healthy choices regarding eating and physical activity which would help overweight or obese children decrease the effects of child obesity.

While childhood obesity may not be prevented by the efforts of school systems alone, schools that have unhealthy environments certainly cause childhood obesity.

The Role of Communities

Environment is a major contributing factor when it comes to influencing childhood obesity. Even community environment is one of the major causes of childhood obesity by shaping the perception and habits of children.

Considering the positive aspects, community environment influences access to healthy and affordable

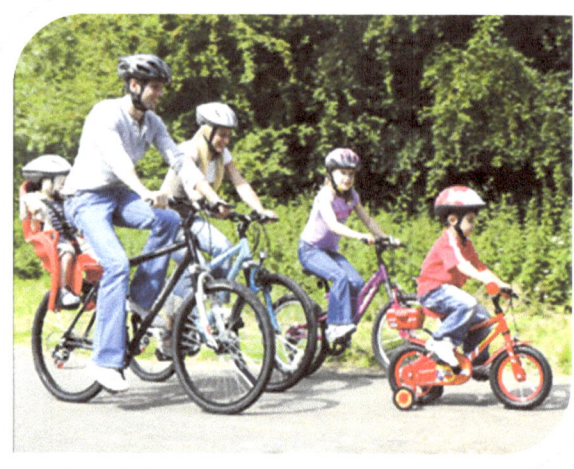

foods as well as physical activity opportunity. For instance, a lack of sidewalks, secure bike and parks in neighbourhoods can discourage children from taking part in physical activities outside their homes or even from walking or biking to school.

Moreover, a lack of healthy food choices and lack of access to affordability in neighbourhood fast food markets can be an obstacle to purchasing healthy foods.

The environmental impact can be measured from the fact that kids get influenced by TV advertisements that promote unhealthy eating habits and foods that contributes greatly into the epidemic of childhood obesity throughout the world. In addition, children are easily influenced within their surrounding environment. Facts that demote the importance of exercise and physical activity.

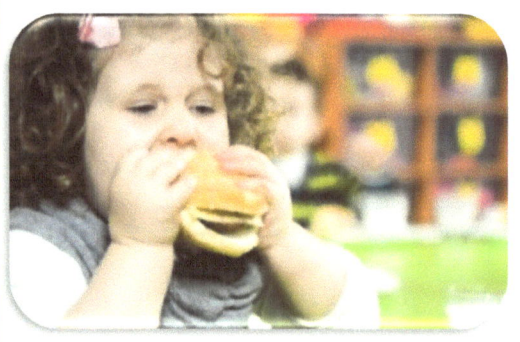

In current terms, it is estimated that approx forty to fifty per cent of every dollar, euro or pound spent on food is basically spent on food outside the home in cafeterias, restaurants and sporting events etc. Moreover, kids also tend to increase the size of their meal especially while eating out as compared to eating at home.

Another negative environmental impact that has taken over children is the consumption of excessive sodas and fruit juices. Such beverages contribute greatly towards child obesity. In fact, a 32 ounce soda contains almost 400 calories, and little children are consuming sodas instead of water.

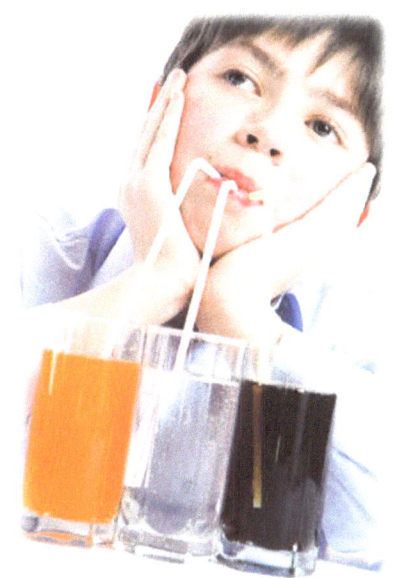

According to scientific studies, when a child consumes a regular soda, he/she becomes 60 per cent more susceptible to obesity threats. Fruit juices, box drinks and sports drinks present another significant problem these days that are being adopted from the environment and communities. The significant amount of calories present in these beverages is estimated to be the major cause of 20 per cent of children who are currently suffering obesity.

Recently lifestyles have made drastic improvements towards the quality of our life but at the same time are contributing towards long term and short term effects. Cars are used for even a walking distance trip while the number of walking trips a child takes each year is decreasing.

Today, only 10 per cent of school students are putting in the effort to walk to school compared to a huge number of students who preferred walking to school and other nearby places than driving, a generation ago. The sedentary lifestyle and the bad food choices are actually adopted from community influence.

There is a significant change the community can make as a whole by contributing towards this great cause of growing childhood obesity. All it requires is sincerity of taking this universal problem as a personal problem and taking all measures to protect our future generations from the threats of childhood obesity.

Read on to find out what efforts you can put in being a community as a whole.

Childhood obesity, in rare cases can be caused by certain medical conditions. These include chemical or hormonal imbalances and inherited disorders of metabolism such as Cushing's syndrome, hypothyroidism, certain neurological problems and even depression that can steer to overeating.

Education levels also contribute to the socio-economic issue associated with childhood obesity. Parents with little or no education are unaware of the severe conditions obesity can lead to. Neither do they have information about proper nutrition and healthy food choices. This makes it difficult to instil those important values in their children.

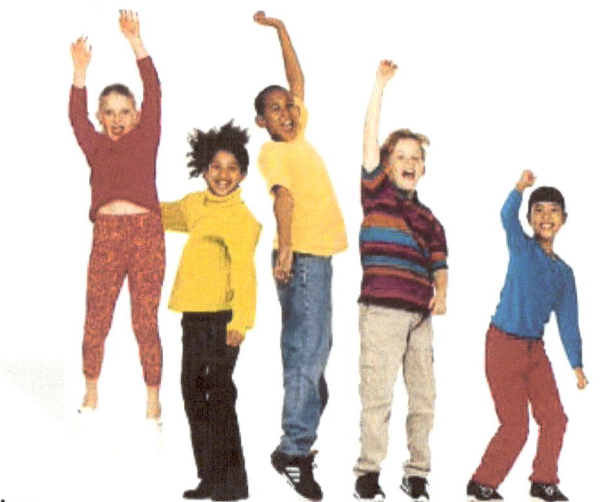

Now that we have discussed all the major contributing factors behind the growing threat of childhood obesity, it's time I disclosed all the preventative measures you can take to avoid childhood obesity.

As you have been reading above – no matter what source is behind childhood obesity – the main reason will always remain the bad eating habits and food choices along with lazy and sedentary lifestyle. Every cause eventually leads to these two major causes and, therefore, the prevention should start from these two causes only.

Therefore, investigate and treat the root factors that are operating behind this growing epidemic and prevent bad eating habits and sedentary lifestyles. The following chapters will educate you step by step in every aspect on how to control childhood obesity from affecting your child. I hope this information will help you in controlling the disastrous effects of childhood obesity. Read on!

Preventing Obesity – Before It's Too Late

It has become a cultural goal to prevent childhood obesity. According to recent statistics, younger population is facing obesity at a higher rate than adult population. Childhood obesity is a real public health problem, accelerating even among toddlers and babies throughout the world.

So what factors should be pondered over that are resulting in childhood obesity? What evidence do we have that suggests that these factors do influence obesity risk? After going through all the factors that are running behind childhood obesity, this part of the book is an effort to find solutions for all those problems and to answer questions as fully as reliable research findings allow.

At a Glance

- Childhood obesity rates are rising at alarming rates and therefore needs to be cured without further delay
- Children who are overweight at the age of three are at the risk of carrying the excessive weight to adulthood as well
- Children learn many of their food choice behaviours from advertisements and their peers instead of what their parents teach them
- According to researchers there are many possible factors that lead to childhood obesity such as genetics, access to fast food items and the lack of child monitoring from parents.

© Oliver Greene

The Role of Parents

"Childhood Obesity Prevention Begins at Home"

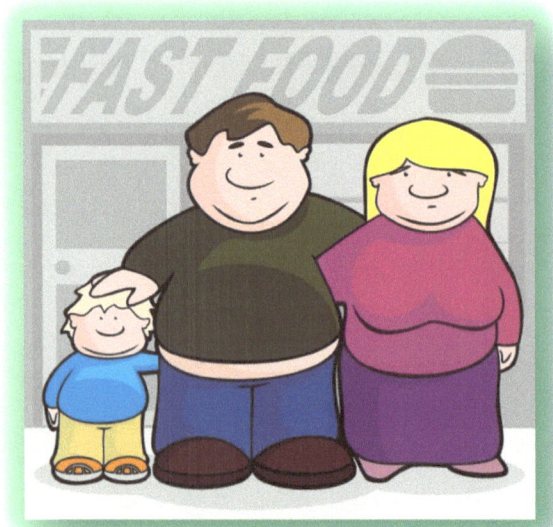

Childhood obesity frequency is highest among children who have two obese parents. Such children are 25 to 30 per cent more likely to become obese like their parents. However, there are cases in which obesity is caused by poor eating habits and family nutrition rather than genetics. It is not easy to segregate genetics from family behavioural and environmental factors as causes of childhood obesity.

The behavioural pattern of a family regarding cooking, shopping, exercising and eating, have a major impact on a child's energy imbalance. It's the responsibility of parents to keep healthy food in access of their children while leaving unhealthy food out of their reach. This is why the entire blame does not fall on your kids for being fascinated by fatty, salty and sweet food – after all you can't deny how tasty this food is.

Most of the children learn their food behaviours in their homes. When they observe that the entire family prefers fast food, hamburgers and processed foods every day, they will be persuaded to follow the same trend and consume unhealthy foods.

In addition, parents having busy schedules pay less attention to the physical activity of their children. In fact, once they are home, they also follow a sedentary and lazy lifestyle which encourages their children to follow the same trend. So what can be done? Let's see!

Studies show that parents are usually their kid's most pivotal role models. Kids who observe their parents living a healthy and active lifestyle are more likely to do the same. As parents, you can take preventative steps that can help your little one prevent child obesity. This chapter has answers that will provide you with plans to help you keep your children active and healthy.

Be a Role Model

Parents play the most important role in their child life. The way you behave helps your child to develop the sense to choose the right food in appropriate quantity and at the perfect time. Moreover, they will also develop the habit of exercising if you stay physically fit and encourage physical activities. This may be challenging at first especially if you are already experiencing a hectic schedule and are busy dealing with the daily life demands.

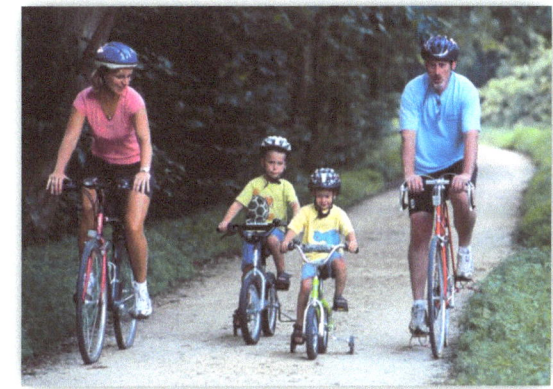

However, if efforts are made collectively, it is likely that you will succeed. Regardless of how difficult changing lifestyle can be at first, gradually healthy habits will become a part of daily routine, which will eventually help in improving the overall health of the family and preventing obesity in children. The following are some suggestions on how parents can be a positive role model for their children.

- Incorporate physical activities in your routine.
- Encourage healthy foods and take time out to prepare food at home instead of going to fast-food restaurants or bringing junk food home.
- Discourage large portion sizes.

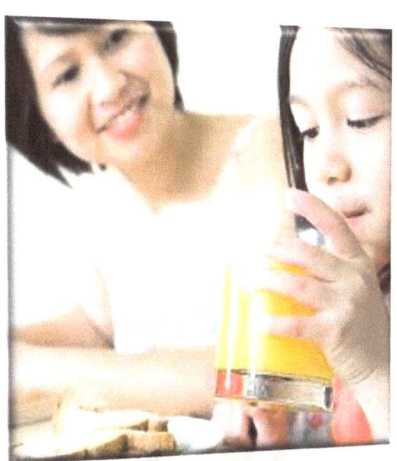

- Dedicate high-calorie foods and sweet treats only for special occasions.
- Engage your children in daily routine activities such as helping you in the kitchen or cleaning their bedrooms instead of allowing them to enjoy extra screen time.
- Pay attention to the importance of adopting healthy lifestyle choices. This will help you more instead of just counting numbers on the scale.

Execute Behavioural Changes to the Entire Family

It will be much easier for the child to adopt behavioural changes if the entire family is following it. This is one of the most efficient ways to prevent childhood obesity. Moreover, developing healthy eating habits and active

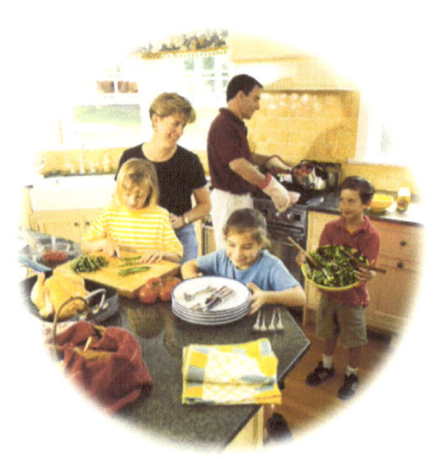

lifestyle will not only affect the children but if adopted by the entire family will help all the family members in the long run.

Balanced changes are easier to adopt and maintain as a part of daily routine. You can start by implementing a few changes in your home. Follow the tips:

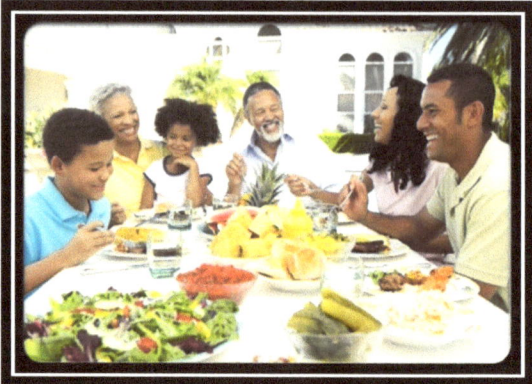

- Observe your child's sleeping routine. Is your child getting sufficient sleep? Make sure your child is sleeping adequately. According to a research held recently, it was concluded that children sleeping extra hours are reducing the risk of obesity by 9%. Children must sleep according to the table below.

Age	Sleeping Hours
5	11 hours or more
6 to 10	10 hours
11 and above	9 hours

- Turn off the Television during meal time. It is always good to limit screen time for children to save them from a lazy lifestyle.
- Encourage children to drink more water or milk instead of soft drinks, fruit juices and sodas.
- Activate family physical activity after dinner. Encourage your family members to clean the table and help to clean in the kitchen. This would give a chance for the calorie intake to turn into energy.

- Assess all the family members, especially the obese ones, and locate reasonable targets for each member and decide on family activity. Set goals such as walking in the park every evening with the entire family and serve fruit salads as evening snacks. Do not forget to add the most important goal of limiting fast food meals in your list.

- Remember! Your child is making an effort to adopt a new lifestyle that restricts him/her from their favourite activities. It is surely more challenging and difficult for your child than it is for you. Therefore, do not forget to pay attention and praise your child whenever you see him/her making an effort. Do not treat them with sweets but fruit.

- Only you can encourage the rest of your family members to play an effective role. Initially, your goal must be to focus on a healthy lifestyle change for your child instead of forcing him/her to lose weight. If you are making too strict aims for your family, consider making amendments. It is always better to switch to a more effective plan that works for everybody instead of a plan that is suitable to only one or two out of all the family members.

You can put efforts to combat childhood obesity at home. The sooner you will

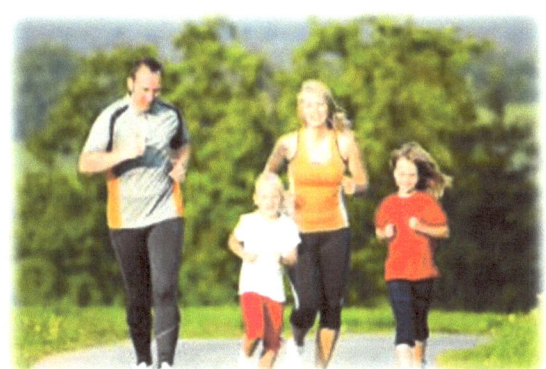

implement the plan and goals, the better. It is much easier to provide a new lifestyle to children than to adults.

Being the fundamental mentor of your child, you must observe and have control over what your child eats. Always make healthy foods, fruits and snacks accessible to your children. Eliminate or minimize fruit juices, sodas and other sweetened beverages as they contain unhealthy ingredients that not only add excessive calories to your child's body but also make your child feel too full to eat healthy foods.

In order to reduce obesity in children, cut down on white carbohydrate intakes such as rice, sugar, bread, pasta and desserts. Maintaining a well-planned meal schedule that follows a strict time-table will encourage children to eat whatever you offer them when they feel hungry. This can turn out to be the first successful step you can take to prevent childhood obesity at home.

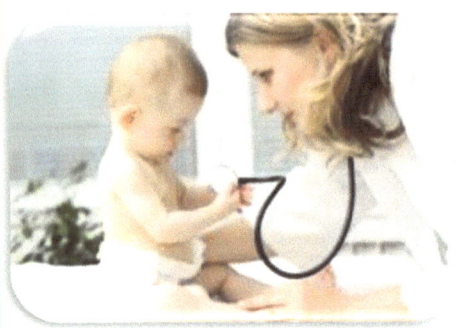

Regardless of your child's age, you can implement the following changes to obtain healthier results.

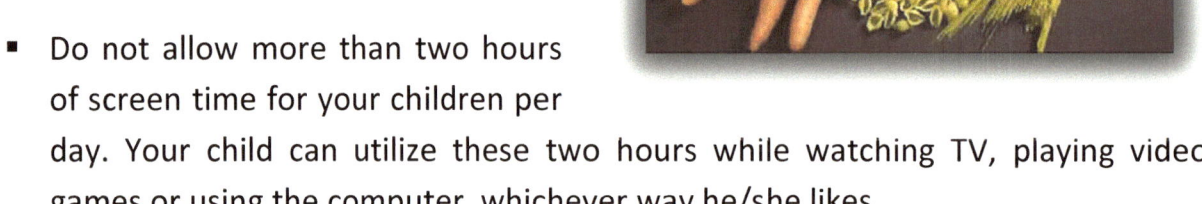

- Do not allow more than two hours of screen time for your children per day. Your child can utilize these two hours while watching TV, playing video games or using the computer, whichever way he/she likes.
- Do not allow your child to eat while watching TV. Most children are so involved in watching TV that they do not pay attention to the portion size of the meal they are eating. This leads to mindless munching that result in excessive eating. Always discourage your child from doing so.
- Offer your children a variety of healthy meals together. This will encourage them to eat homemade healthy food.
- Offer your children at least 5 servings of vegetables and fruit per day. This will provide sufficient nutrition their body requires.
- Make sure your children are regularly eating their healthy breakfast every day.

Being the parents, you must also take proactive measures to ensure whether or not your child is suffering through obesity threats or not.

Seek medical Assistance

Take the help of your doctor and schedule a visit to the doctor. It is important for you to understand the growth of your child. The doctor will start of by finding the BMI of your child. Even if it does not cross the obesity parameters, an increase in your child's BMI over a year is an indication that your child may be at the risk of obesity.

Do not encourage your child with food rewards

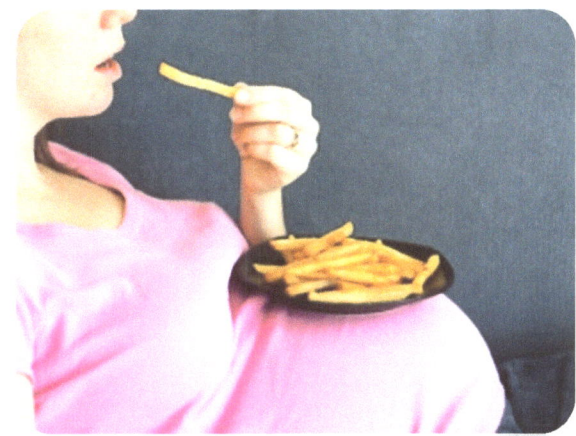

Do not encourage any of your child's acts with food rewards. In short, food items such as candies and fast food meals should not be used for behaviour modification in children. Instead, it can result in an adverse impact.

Positive behaviour should be encouraged

Encourage your child while he/she adopts the new lifestyle laid down by you. Make it fun rather than a hectic plan or job that needs to be done. Be a part of it and enjoy every moment with your child while he/she is putting in effort to revitalize himself/herself. Pay attention and observe your child and never let him/her fall back. Remember. Your children seek your encouragement.

Bottom-line

Many obese and overweight children grow and carry additional weight to adulthood. Therefore, it is very important to prevent your child from becoming obese at a very early age. Controlling childhood obesity can even start from when you child is a fetus. Don't believe it? Then read the next chapter!

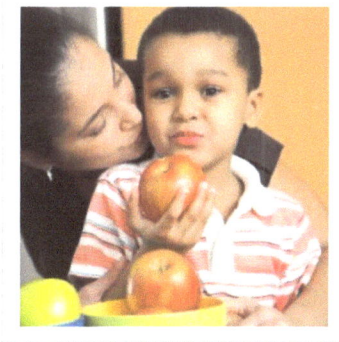

Pregnant Moms- Are You Carrying An Obese Fetus?

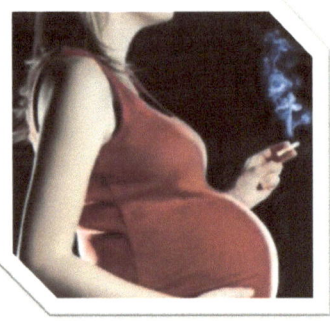

According to a recent study, it has been discovered that the reason why pregnant women are carrying an obese fetus is the fact that during pregnancy, women eat for both herself and the baby. It is warned, pregnant women should not eat for two. Women who gain extra weight in pregnancy put both themselves and their unborn babies at risk, as well as increase the risk of over-weight health problems in later life.

This was further studied in depth, concluding that the excessive weight gained during pregnancy is not only dangerous to the life of the mother but also for the child. Women follow the myth of eating for two as the baby requires additional food. This is not true. The baby is fed on whatever the mom eats and a single person's food is quite sufficient even when the woman is expecting at month six.

The first six months of pregnancy, women should stick to their recommended intake of around 1950 calories each day. Following the wrong approach, almost half of expectant mothers are obese or overweight putting themselves at a much higher risk of fatal health conditions such as pre-eclampsia, blood clots, still births and even miscarriages.

Overeating not only results in obese pregnant mom but also obese fetus that eventually becomes an obese baby.

There are many factors related to the risk of obesity in infancy and early childhood. These factors include smoking during gestation, unnecessary maternal weight gain,

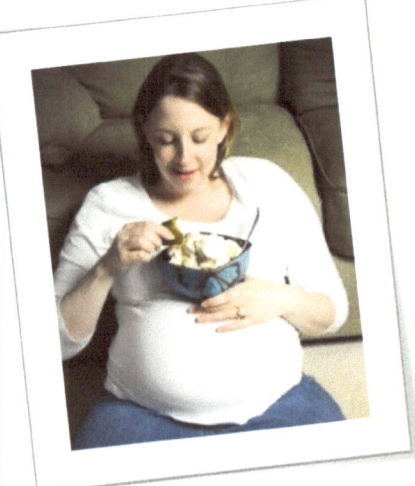

suboptimal sleeping durations during infancy and less than recommended breast-feeding duration. During the development procedure of a baby inside and outside the womb, such exposures result in long-term regulation of energy imbalance that eventually results in increased risk of childhood obesity.

These exposures usually persuade the formation of endocrine pancreatic function and hypothalamic circuits that regulate body weight. In short, it disturbs the entire cycle of metabolic programming.

In order to control your unborn baby's weight, mothers must quit smoking during pregnancy and should not put on excessive weight. Moreover, they should increase the duration of breast-feed as well as increase the sleep duration according to adequate timing. These interventions should be included in a comprehensive obesity-prevention effort, since it has a life-long childhood obesity risk associated with it.

If early interventions are applied, it will definitely prevent the growth of obesity and other health issues in school children. Many health campaigns are contributing towards achieving the aim of extending the period of breast feeding in mothers as well as conducting programs that help mothers to quit smoking. Efforts are also being made to address the problem of excessive weight gain during pregnancy.

By understanding the life threatening risks of life-long obesity that starts to develop in infancy and early childhood, mothers can play an important role in reversing the overall impact of childhood obesity epidemic.

Prevention through Education

Education can be a very powerful tool in preventing obesity, since it can serve as one of the most fundamental agents in addressing the childhood obesity crisis. In fact, education and schools can have 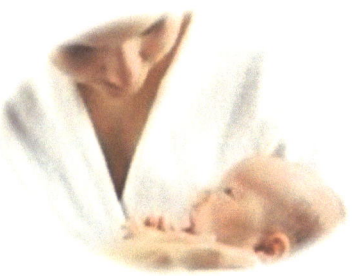 both positive and negative impacts on childhood obesity. We have already discussed how life and unhealthy meal plans at school are becoming one of the major causes behind childhood obesity. On the other hand, many schools are creating new school health policies to prevent childhood obesity.

According to The Institute of Medicine, many schools are increasingly implementing different health programs that focus on increasing physical activity and improving the nutrition of students.

Increased Opportunities for Students to Engage In Physical Activities and Sports

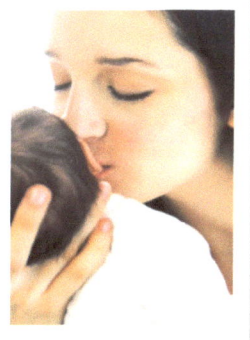

The policymakers of different schools are now beginning to understand the importance of physical education for school children. They are accepting the fact that physical education is an important part of academic discipline and must be taught in school. This is the discipline that teaches students the most critical skills required to become a productive citizen of the 21st century.

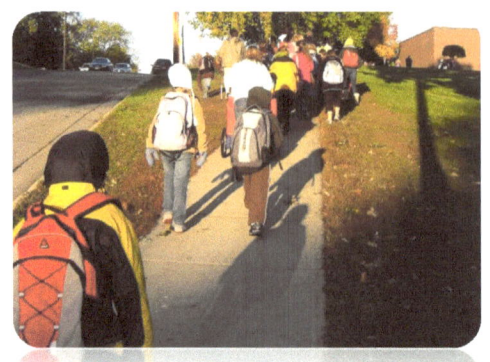

Many schools are now offering different opportunities to benefit from physical activity in after-school programs, in-school programs, activities outside of physical education class in physical activity clubs as well as during recess periods for free-form play in elementary schools.

The opportunity is offered to everybody equally. Surprisingly, many teachers are promoting health education to such an extent that they are offering students opportunities for physical education in the classroom as a part of planned lessons that teach them language arts, mathematics and several other academic concepts through movement.

Another very important approach is to encourage students to walk to school. While this was the norm of most students a few years ago, walking to school rarely exists now. In

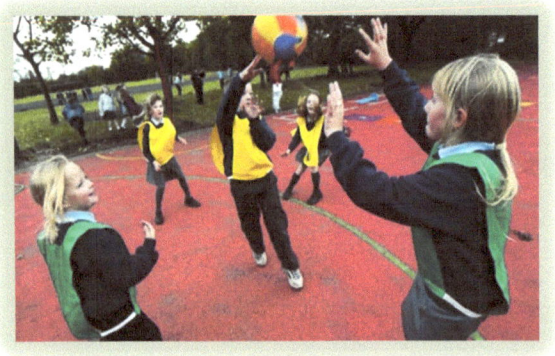

fact, more than 2/3 of students who reside even a mile away do not prefer walking to school. The International Walk to School Day was an important step taken to promote walking to school once again. Many communities are established to ensure that children are using the safe routes to school so that they do not face any barriers to walking.

Schools are offering a combination of physical activities for children such as recreation, team sports, swimming and running. Implementing an active lifestyle in school gives courage to overweight or obese children in fighting emotional and psychological damage caused by childhood obesity.

Moreover, emphasis on physical education also helps children learn how to cope with obesity caused by traumatic events such as social ridicule, abuse and low self-esteem. It also teaches children worthwhile skills that can be implemented throughout their lives, such as healthy eating habits and teamwork.

Implement a Quality School Meal Program

Schools are an ideal setting for the implementation of healthy eating habits. In fact, many schools are putting in an effort to create various programs with that aim. This is because school is the place where a child spends most hours of the day and adopts behaviour that surrounds him or her.

To bring changes to the lifestyle of the students considering the obesity menace, schools should make an array of changes to the nutrition policy to prevent obesity. The changes can be like replacing soda with low-fat milk, water or 100% fruit juice. Schools

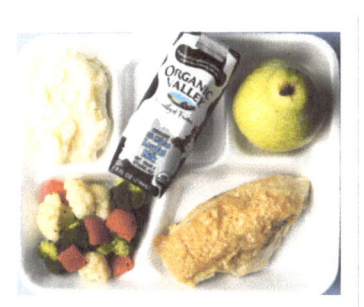 should also discourage the idea of having cafeterias with snacks, fast foods and vending machines that do not meet certain nutrition criteria. Schools must also make an effort 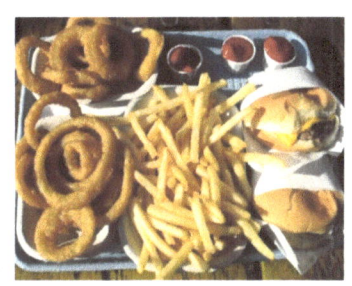 to educate children on how exercise and diet affect their health and make them active.

Nutrition education is vital. It gives students the sense of determination they require in order to make healthy food choices which eventually encourage and help them decrease threats of childhood obesity.

Schools can also involve parents through nutrition workshops and meetings that persuade them to provide their children with more healthy food such as vegetables and fruit. Involving parents is a good step towards preventing childhood obesity because after school hours children are under the supervision of their parents. If similar strategies are used at home and in school, it will become easier for the child to settle in.

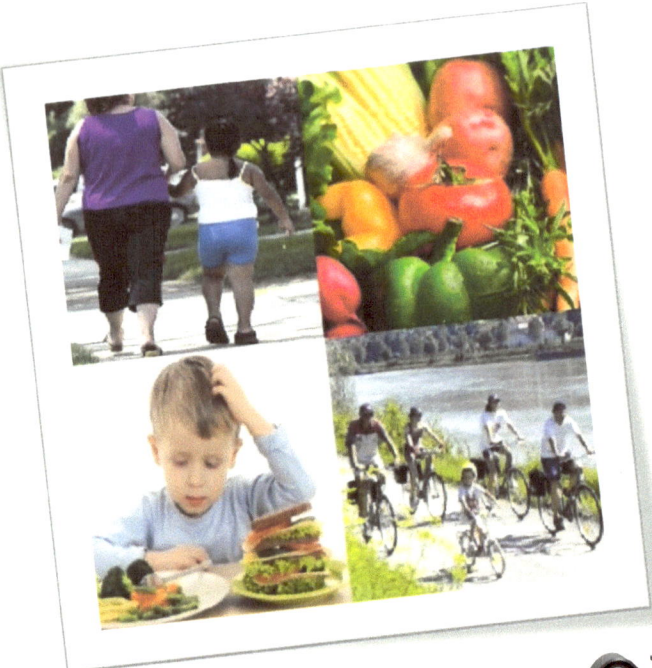

According to studies, school lunches can still be served to a better standard to students. There are many essential nutrients missing from school lunches, however. Certain ingredients like salt are usually excessive. No matter how 'yummy' the meal in the right picture above is for your child, the left picture is the perfect example of a healthy lunch at school. Not only does it have a bit of everything, it also has almost all nutrients that your child needs. Moreover, the left plate has paid attention to every little thing that many schools overlook for example low-fat milk that is recommended by dieticians and paediatricians. The plate also has the appropriate serving of fruit and salad.

OR

To sum up, without a strong contribution from schools, the childhood obesity epidemic is unlikely to reverse.

Choosing a Strategy – Diet or Exercise? BOTH!!!

From the beginning of this book, one thing is quite clear. Prevention of obesity depends on two major factors – improved eating habits and non-sedentary lifestyle. Depending on a single factor will not be as productive as considering both factors together. Being a parent, it is very important for you to teach your children the ABC's of life. Especially,

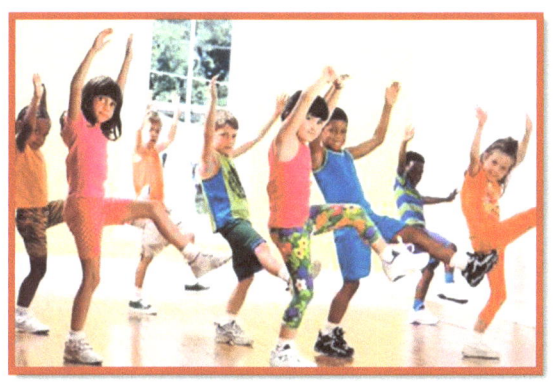 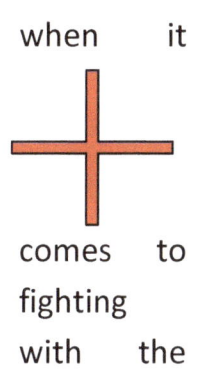 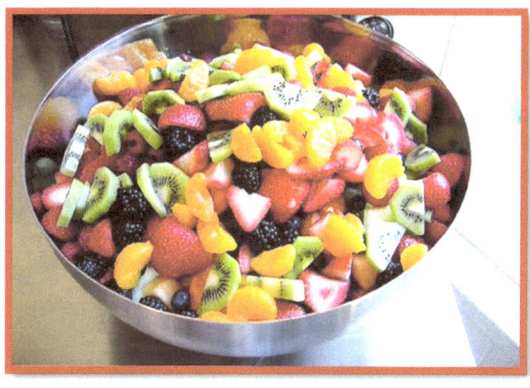

when it comes to fighting with the growing epidemic of childhood obesity and adopting healthy eating habits and active lifestyle, the 'ABCDE' of life is essential. So tell your child it's high time that he/she should

"Act Boldly to Change Diet and Exercise"
"ABCDE"

The Importance

High-quality nutrition and lots of exercise are the building blocks for healthy development, strong growth, and life-long wellbeing for children. The reason why obesity is rapidly increasing in children is that most of them are not receiving the adequate amount of nutrition and exercise regularly. This is because:

a) Children do not eat enough fruit and vegetables
b) Children do not eat enough HEALTHY meals
c) Children are not getting enough exercise

The Benefits of Good Nutrition and Regular Exercise for Children

Behavioural and Mental State

- High-quality nutrition is indispensable to the development of healthy brain in children, which is definitely critical to learning.
- Children who are provided with healthy nutrition are likely to:

I.   Show great academic performance

II.   Feel confident about themselves, their looks and their capabilities

III.   Avoid depression, anxiety and low-self esteem

IV.   Absorb stress and tackle with their emotions in a much better way

- Adopting a healthy lifestyle at an early age will help your child to lead a healthy and active life in the long run.

Physical Benefits

- Children's metabolisms are different and therefore require different combinations of nutrients such as complex carbs, proteins, healthy fats, vitamins and minerals. These nutrients help children in development and growth and save them from different illnesses.

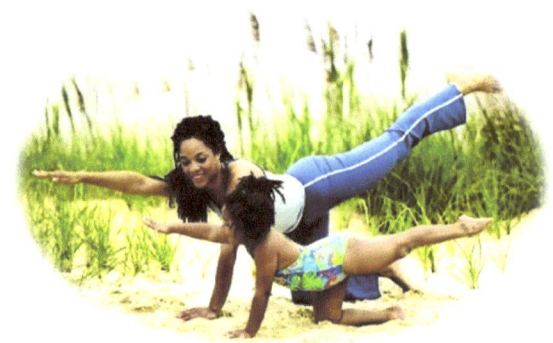

- Regular exercise helps children to build stronger bones and muscles along with limiting excessive body fat.

- Healthy eating helps in managing eating disorders, eliminate risk of cavities, iron deficiency, malnutrition and also cuts down on unhealthy weight control behaviours, i.e. skipping meals, fasting, eating insufficient amount of food, using diet pills, vomiting, diuretics and laxatives.

- Regular physical activities and healthy eating help to control persistent diseases that appear in adulthood associated with obesity. These include type2 diabetes, heart disease, different types of cancer and high blood pressure.

Instinctively, children try to copy their parents in every way. This is why it is always recommended that parents enforce changes in themselves before they try to implement them on their children. Now that you know that you exert the most impact on your children's behaviour, it is time that you make the most out of it. Become the ideal of your children and model healthy habits and attitudes towards physical activity and food to influence your children to do the same.

Moreover, you also hold the control of the types of food your children can access at home. Make sure you minimize the access to unhealthy food and make a space so that your children welcome healthy, wholesome foods such as vegetables, fruits, whole grains, lean proteins and low fat dairy.

Do not forget to monitor your children's daily routine. Limit or eliminate everything you do not consider appropriate for your child's health, but slowly and gradually. Have patience and give time to your children to open up their mind for the new change so that they accept it happily. Educate your children about living healthy lifestyles and complement them whenever they take a step ahead. However, make sure you do not complement them by giving them a sweet treat!

The Perfect Weekly Fitness - Table for Your Child

Now here is the most ideal health-table you can set for your child. It will help you construct a proper plan. You are most welcome to make amendments according to the likes and dislikes of your child. But make sure you do not add any unhealthy ingredient to this healthy mix-plate. Here it goes:

Cut Down On

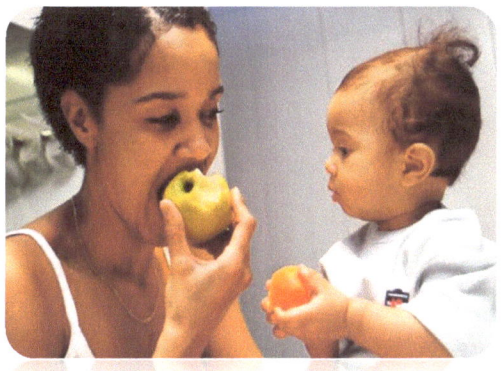

Excessive TV watching or playing games on TV or computer. Also cut down on inactive sitting for a very long time.

This may exhaust your child because even though he/she has leisure time available, they are unable to spend it playing video games or watching TV at home. This will encourage them to move out of the house and play with other children and get some physical activity. Good start right?

2-3 Times Per Week

Playtime and Leisure
Canoeing
Swinging
Tumbling
Miniature Golf

Flexibility and Strength
Martial Arts
pull-ups/push-ups
Rope Climbing
Dancing

This two to three week health routine has options for both girls and boys. Mentioned earlier are some of the most effective physical activities that help the children to stay fit and maintain healthy energy balance.

3-5 Times Per Week

Aerobic Exercise (min 20 minutes)
Swimming
Biking
Rope Climbing
Running
Skateboarding

Outdoor Activities (min 20 minutes)
Basketball
Kickball
Volleyball
Racing
Soccer

Mentioned above are the most well known indoor and outdoor activities that are a great source of healthy physical activity. Children can choose to play basketball or soccer outdoors with friends or can choose to stay indoors and swim. In any case, only twenty minutes every day can bring great changes to their lifestyles.

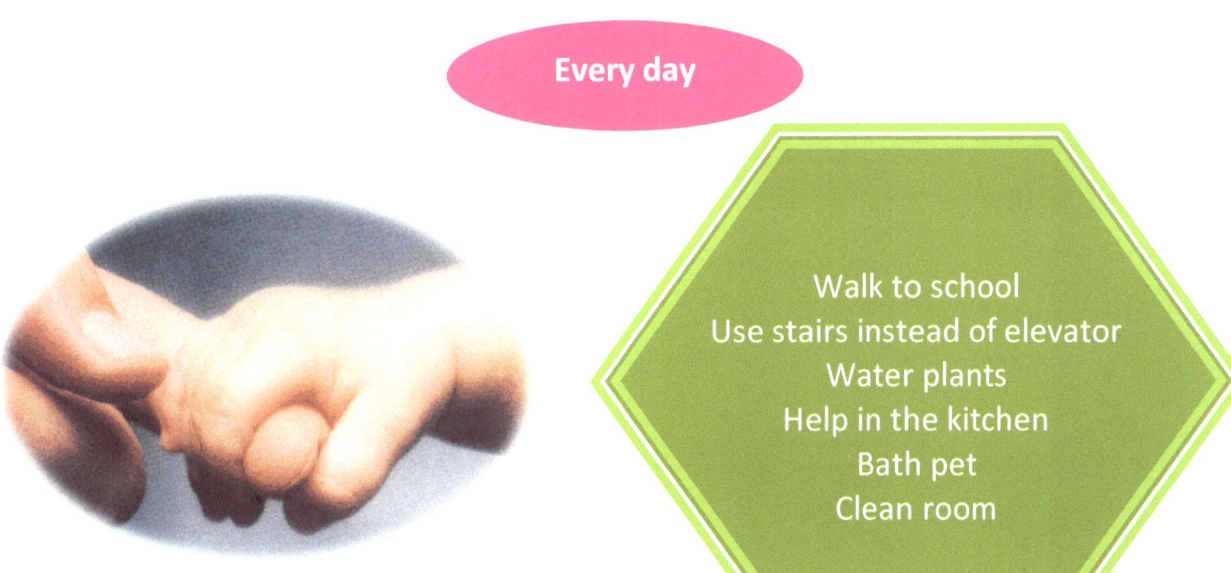

Every day

Walk to school
Use stairs instead of elevator
Water plants
Help in the kitchen
Bath pet
Clean room

These are the most common things you can add to your children's routine. Not only does it help develop good habits, it also helps cut down obesity risks.

Be Your Children's Best Friend

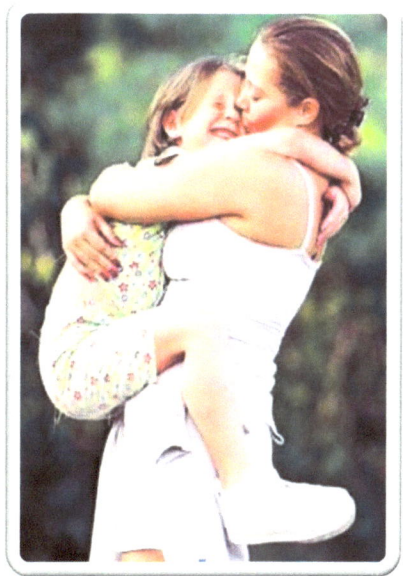

Do you know your child is at risk of becoming obese? Do you realize who does he/she needs the most right now? **YOU**! Being parents or caregivers, your child will count on you the most to give him/her the courage and moral support they need and to pull him/her out of this growing epidemic of childhood obesity.

You are indeed your children's best friend. Treat them well. Tell them you will turn everything perfect. If you are not an obese parent, perhaps you will not be able to understand the current mental state of your children. Obesity makes a person feel as if he/she is different from rest of the world and can never look handsome or beautiful.

Too emotional right? Make it fun! After all those physical activities mix-plate mentioned earlier, it's time to make a real mix-plate of nutritious food for your children. Create the magic in your kitchen this time. I have gathered some delicious and highly nutritious recipes for your children. Try them and your children will love you.

Creamy Avocado-Broccoli Soup

Ingredients

Few broccoli flowers
1 medium size avocado
1 red or green pepper
1 onion (yellow)
1 celery stalk
Salt according to taste
2 cups of yeast free vegetable broth
Basil, cumin, fresh cilantro and other spices of your choice

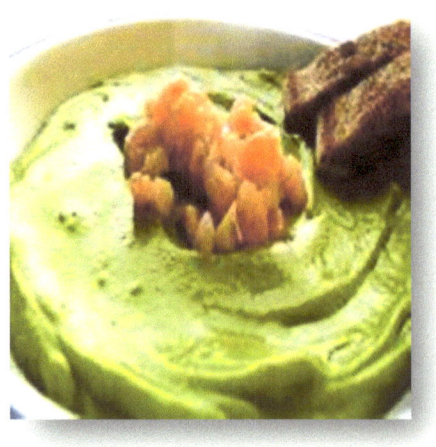

How to Prepare:

Heat vegetable broth and add chopped onion and broccoli and warm for several minutes. Add avocado, pepper and celery in a blender and blend until the puree becomes soup and creamy (add water if desired). Flavour with your favourite spices and serve warm.

Grapefruit-Carrot Shake

Ingredients

2 carrots
1 Grapefruit
3 oz. pure water
3 ice cubes

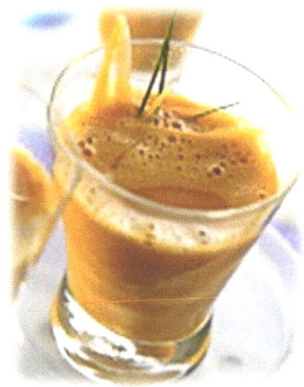

2-3 mint leaves

How to Prepare:

First, peel the grapefruit and push the grapefruit through the juicer, collecting juice in cup. Then wash the carrots, trim off the ends and also push through juicer. Pour both juices into a tall glass, add the water and mix well. Finally add the ice cubes and decorate with mint leaves.

Vegetable Pasta with Tomato-Pepper Sauce

Ingredients

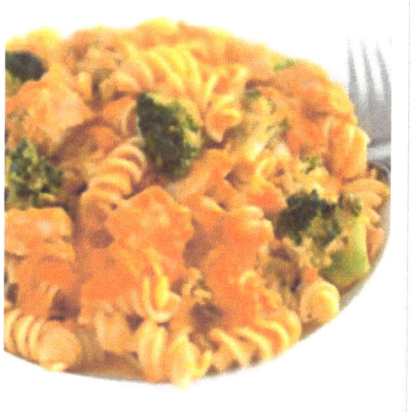

500g vegetable or spelt pasta
300g tomatoes
½ cup sun dried tomatoes
1 small red bell pepper
1 small zucchini
1 onion
2 garlic cloves
1 chilli
5 fresh basil leaves
2-3 tbsp. cold-pressed olive oil
Salt and pepper to taste

How to Prepare:

Cook vegetable or spelt pasta according to directions. Cut tomatoes, bell pepper and zucchini in cubes and finely chop onion, garlic and chilli. Heat olive oil in pan. Add onion, pepper, chili and garlic, and fry for a couple of minutes. Then add the tomatoes and zucchini and cook for approximately 5-10 minutes. Lastly, add the basil and taste with pepper and salt. Put pasta on plate, top with sauce and garnish if desired.

Super Soy Pudding

Ingredients

1 cup fresh almond milk
2 avocados
Juice of 1 lime
2 scoops of Soy Powder
1 pkg. Stevia
6-8 ice cubes

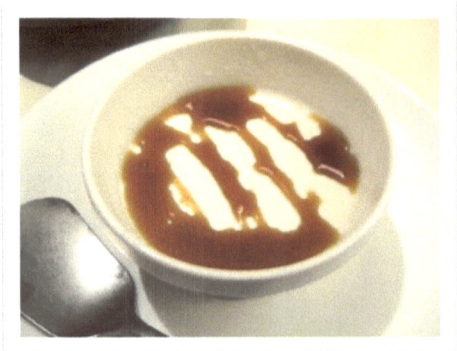

How to Prepare:

Put all ingredients in a blender and mix until the pudding is smooth and pudding-like. Enjoy this healthy dessert!

Grilled Veggies

Ingredients

1 big zucchini
1 big eggplant
1 red bell pepper
1 yellow bell pepper
1 green bell pepper
4 carrots
1 big onion
2 cloves of garlic
3 tbsp. olive oil
Fresh herbs, e.g. oregano, thyme, basil
Salt and freshly ground pepper

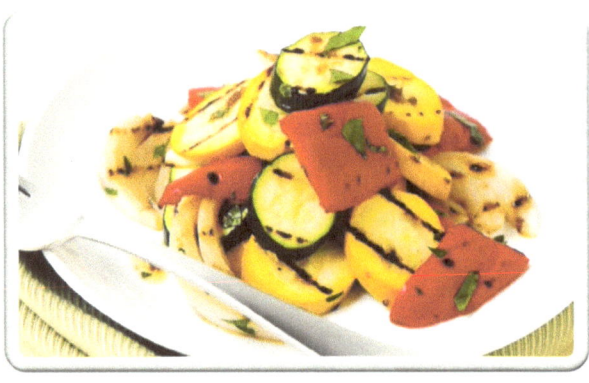

How to Prepare:

Preheat oven to 350°F (180°C). Dice eggplant, zucchini and bell peppers to bite-sized pieces. Cut the carrots and the onion into fine slices, and crush the garlic. Place all veggies in a big bowl, add the olive oil and mix well, so that all veggies are coated lightly. Now place the veggies onto a baking tray. Season with salt and pepper and sprinkle the freshly chopped herbs over the vegetables. Grill the veggies at 325°F (180°C) for 20-30 minutes.

These are a few recipes to get you started. So do give it a try. Your children will definitely love it!

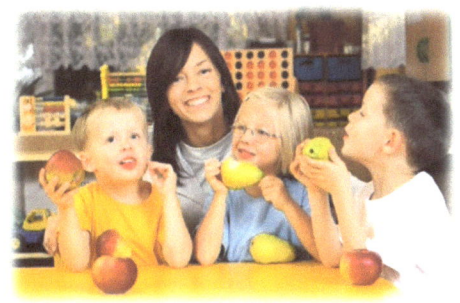

Conclusion

So finally when I am concluding this book, it is time for you to begin. Certainly, saving your child from the menace of obesity is in your own hands. You just need to pay attention and give this issue time.

You can get another job, another car even another house. But you can't get the most precious part of your life back once you lose them – your children! Don't take childhood obesity lightly. The threats are real and so are the facts. The current population of children is the most obese ever in the history of the world.

Although much effort is required on your part, you can't deny the quote, "united we stand, divided we fall". Therefore, the change should be promoted individually and as a family. All families who are affected by this growing epidemic should make collective efforts to fight childhood obesity.

Childhood obesity is a global problem and if you play your role in saving your children from this growing epidemic, you will be contributing towards a major cause.

So understand your responsibility and don't ignore the facts. It is indeed a matter of life and death. Your efforts today can give your child a beautiful and healthy future. All you need to do is take the time to dedicate yourself to your children. When you succeed in helping your child, you will know your effort was worth it!

We have endeavoured to help you and your children avoid obesity. Please do not let child obesity destroy a life.
We wish you every success in your daily life.

Should you require any further help please e-mail me oliver@the-menace-of-obesity.com

Other Books by Oliver Greene

Obesity Worldwide

ISBN 978-1-910053-70-6

The Menace Of Obesity

ISBN 978-1-4568 89920

The Encyclopedia of Herbs

Fruits & Vegetables

ISBN 978-1-4568-80044